KT-364-806

Contents

Introduction

COMPLEMENTARY MEDICINE is Volume 343 in the **ISSUES** series. The aim of the series is to offer current, diverse information about important issues in our world, from a UK perspective.

ABOUT COMPLEMENTARY MEDICINE

Herbal medicines, acupuncture, yoga and 'giggle doctors' are just a few of the complementary and alternative medicines and therapies available today. This book explores the many treatments which are on offer to patients. It also considers the safety and effectiveness of using them.

OUR SOURCES

Titles in the **ISSUES** series are designed to function as educational resource books, providing a balanced overview of a specific subject.

The information in our books is comprised of facts, articles and opinions from many different sources, including:

⇨ Newspaper reports and opinion pieces

⇨ Website factsheets

⇨ Magazine and journal articles

⇨ Statistics and surveys

⇨ Government reports

⇨ Literature from special interest groups.

A NOTE ON CRITICAL EVALUATION

Because the information reprinted here is from a number of different sources, readers should bear in mind the origin of the text and whether the source is likely to have a particular bias when presenting information (or when conducting their research). It is hoped that, as you read about the many aspects of the issues explored in this book, you will critically evaluate the information presented.

It is important that you decide whether you are being presented with facts or opinions. Does the writer give a biased or unbiased report? If an opinion is being expressed, do you agree with the writer? Is there potential bias to the 'facts' or statistics behind an article?

ASSIGNMENTS

In the back of this book, you will find a selection of assignments designed to help you engage with the articles you have been reading and to explore your own opinions. Some tasks will take longer than others and there is a mixture of design, writing and research-based activities that you can complete alone or in a group.

Useful weblinks

www.1023.org.uk

www.cancerresearchuk.org

www.derby.ac.uk

www.gov.uk

www.ibtimes.co.uk

www.independent.co.uk

www.indigo-herbs.co.uk

www.macmillan.org.uk

www.medicalnewstoday.com

www.nhs.uk

www.nimh.org.uk

www.nutritionist-resource.org.uk

www.telegraph.co.uk

www.theconversation.com

www.theguardian.com

www.therapy-directory.org.uk

www.rchm.co.uk

FURTHER RESEARCH

At the end of each article we have listed its source and a website that you can visit if you would like to conduct your own research. Please remember to critically evaluate any sources that you consult and consider whether the information you are viewing is accurate and unbiased.

Complementary Medicine

Editor: Tina Brand

Volume 343

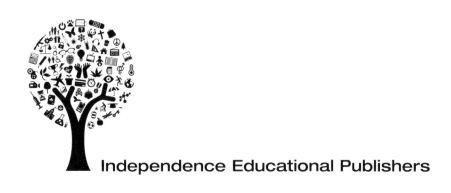

Independence Educational Publishers

First published by Independence Educational Publishers

The Studio, High Green

Great Shelford

Cambridge CB22 5EG

England

Copyright

Photocopy licence

ISBN-13: 978 1 86168 794 4

Printed in Great Britain

Zenith Print Group

The difference between complementary and alternative therapies (CAMs)

There is an important difference between a complementary therapy and an alternative therapy.

The phrases 'complementary therapy' and 'alternative therapy' are often used as if they mean the same thing. They may also be combined into one phrase – complementary and alternative therapies (CAMs).

A complementary therapy means you can use it alongside your conventional medical treatment. It may help you to feel better and cope better with your cancer and treatment.

An alternative therapy is generally used instead of conventional medical treatment.

All conventional cancer treatments, such as chemotherapy and radiotherapy, have to go through rigorous testing by law in order to prove that they work. Most alternative therapies have not been through such testing and there is no scientific evidence that they work. Some types of alternative therapy may not be completely safe and could cause harmful side effects.

What are complementary therapies?

Complementary therapies are used alongside conventional medical treatments prescribed by your doctor. They can help people with cancer to feel better and may improve your quality of life. They may also help you to cope better with symptoms caused by the cancer or side effects caused by cancer treatment.

A good complementary therapist won't claim that the therapy will cure your cancer. They will always encourage you to discuss any therapies with your cancer doctor or GP.

There are many different types of complementary therapy, including:

⇨ aromatherapy

⇨ acupuncture

⇨ herbal medicine

⇨ massage therapy

⇨ visualisation

⇨ yoga.

Many health professionals are supportive of people with cancer using complementary therapies. There are some health professionals that have been reluctant for their patients to use them. This is usually because many therapies have not been scientifically tested in the same way as conventional treatments.

Research has been carried out to see how well complementary therapies work for people with cancer. And there is some still in progress. But we need more to find out how best to use complementary therapies.

What are alternative therapies?

Alternative therapies are used instead of conventional medical treatment. People with cancer have various reasons for wanting to try alternative therapies.

There is no scientific or medical evidence to show that alternative therapies can cure cancer. Some alternative therapies are unsafe and can cause harmful side effects. Or they may interact with your conventional medical treatment. This could increase the risk of harmful side effects or may stop the conventional treatment working so well. Giving up your conventional cancer treatment could reduce your chance of curing or controlling your cancer.

Some alternative therapies sound promising but the claims are not supported by scientific evidence and can give some people false hope.

Examples of alternative cancer therapies include:

⇨ laetrile

⇨ shark cartilage

⇨ Gerson therapy.

Other terms used to describe CAM therapies

There are several different terms commonly used to describe complementary or alternative therapies. If you're not familiar with them, it can be confusing. You may see therapies described as:

Unconventional therapies

This generally means treatments that aren't normally used by doctors to treat cancer. In other words, any treatment that is not thought of as part of conventional medicine.

CAM (Complementary and Alternative Medicine)

CAM is a term which covers both complementary and alternative medical therapies.

Integrated healthcare or integrated medicine

These terms are generally used to describe the use of conventional medicine and complementary therapies together. The terms are commonly used in the USA but are becoming more widely used in the UK.

In cancer care, integrated medicine usually includes making sure that you have access to all of the following:

⇨ conventional medical treatments

⇨ different types of complementary therapies such as massage, reflexology, relaxation, herbal medicine and acupuncture

⇨ counselling services and support groups

⇨ up-to-date information about your cancer and its treatment.

Traditional medicine

Health professionals usually use the term 'traditional medicine' to mean a therapy or health practice that has developed over centuries within a particular culture. It's usually formed around a particular belief system.

This term can be confusing because in the western part of the world conventional medicine could be considered to be a traditional medicine. But this term is not usually used in this way. It generally refers to therapies or treatments that developed in the eastern part of the world such as Ayurvedic medicine and traditional Chinese medicine.

26 February 2018

⇨ The above content is supplied by the world's largest charitable funder of cancer research, Cancer Research UK. Please visit www.cancerresearchuk.org for further information.

Osteopathy

Osteopathy is a way of detecting, treating and preventing health problems by moving, stretching and massaging a person's muscles and joints.

Osteopathy is based on the principle that the well-being of an individual depends on their bones, muscles, ligaments and connective tissue functioning smoothly together.

Osteopaths use physical manipulation, stretching and massage with the aim of:

⇨ increasing the mobility of joints

⇨ relieving muscle tension

⇨ enhancing the blood supply to tissues

⇨ helping the body to heal.

They use a range of techniques, but not drugs or surgery.

In the UK, osteopathy is a health profession regulated by UK law.

Although osteopaths may use some conventional medical techniques, the use of osteopathy isn't always based on scientific evidence.

Common uses

Most people who see an osteopath do so for help with conditions that affect the muscles, bones and joints, such as:

⇨ lower back pain

⇨ uncomplicated neck pain (as opposed to neck pain after an injury such as whiplash)

⇨ shoulder pain and elbow pain (for example, tennis elbow)

⇨ arthritis

⇨ problems with the pelvis, hips and legs

⇨ sports injuries

⇨ muscle and joint pain associated with driving, work or pregnancy.

Some osteopaths claim to be able to treat conditions that aren't directly related to muscles, bones and joints, such as headaches, migraines, painful periods, digestive disorders, depression and excessive crying in babies (colic).

But there isn't enough evidence to suggest that osteopathy can treat these problems.

Does osteopathy work?

The National Institute for Health and Care Excellence (NICE) recommends manual therapy alongside exercise as a treatment option for lower back pain, with or without sciatica.

There's limited evidence to suggest that osteopathy may be effective for some types of neck, shoulder or lower-limb pain, and recovery after hip or knee operations.

There's currently no good evidence that it's effective as a treatment for health conditions unrelated to the bones and muscles (musculoskeletal system).

Accessing osteopathy

While osteopathy isn't widely available on the NHS, your GP or local clinical commissioning group (CCG) should be able to tell you whether it's available in your area.

Most people pay for osteopathy treatment privately. Treatment costs vary, but typically range from £35 to £50 for a 30- to 40-minute session.

You don't need to be referred by your GP to see an osteopath privately. Most private health insurance providers also provide cover for osteopathic treatment.

Only people registered with the General Osteopathic Council (GOsC) are allowed to practise as or call themselves osteopaths.

How it's performed

During your first osteopathy session, the osteopath will ask about your symptoms, general health and any other medical care you're receiving before carrying out a physical examination.

The osteopath will use their hands to find areas of weakness, tenderness, restriction or strain within your body, particularly the spine.

With your consent, you'll probably need to remove some clothing from the area being examined, and you may be asked to perform simple movements.

You should then be able to discuss whether osteopathy can help treat the problem and, if so, what the treatment programme should involve.

Osteopaths are trained to identify when a patient needs to be referred to a GP or needs further tests, such as MRI scans or blood tests, to help diagnose the problem.

Osteopathic techniques

An osteopath aims to restore the normal function and stability of the joints to help the body heal itself.

They use their hands to treat your body in a variety of ways, using a mixture of gentle and forceful techniques.

Techniques are chosen based on the individual patient and the symptoms they have reported.

These include:

⇨ massage – to release and relax muscles

⇨ stretching stiff joints

⇨ articulation – where your joints are moved through their natural range of motion

⇨ high-velocity thrusts – short, sharp movements to the spine, which normally produce a clicking noise similar to cracking your knuckles.

These techniques aim to reduce pain, improve movement and encourage blood flow.

Osteopathy isn't usually painful, although it's not unusual to feel sore or stiff in the first few days after treatment, particularly if you're having treatment for a painful or inflamed injury.

Your osteopath will explain whether you're likely to have any reactions. If you feel any pain during or after treatment, tell your osteopath.

You may be given advice on self-help and exercise to aid your recovery and prevent symptoms returning or getting worse.

In general, the first appointment will last about 45 minutes to an hour. Further treatments last around 30 minutes. Your course of treatment will depend on your symptoms.

Osteopathy is a regulated health profession that's distinct from nursing, medicine and pharmacy.

Regulation works in much the same way as regulation for medical doctors.

Regulation

By law, osteopaths must be registered with the General Osteopathic Council (GOsC).

The GOsC only accepts registration from practitioners who have a qualification in osteopathy that's recognised by the GOsC and who comply with their standards of practice.

Osteopaths are required to renew their registration each year. As part of this process, the GOsC checks they have the correct insurance, are meeting professional development requirements, and remain in good health.

If you use an osteopath and they don't adhere to this standard of practice, you can complain to the GOsC. It has a duty to investigate the complaint.

The GOsC has a register of osteopaths you can use to find one in your local area.

Regulation aims to protect patient safety, but it doesn't mean there's scientific evidence that a treatment is effective.

What qualifications do osteopaths have?

Osteopaths complete a four- or five-year honours degree programme (bachelor's or master's), which involves at least 1,000 hours of clinical training. Some osteopaths are qualified to PhD level.

Safety

Osteopathy is generally regarded as a safe treatment, although you may experience minor side effects, such as:

⇨ mild to moderate soreness or pain in the treatment area

⇨ headache

⇨ fatigue

These effects usually develop within a few hours of a session and typically get better on their own within a day or two.

In rare cases, serious complications have been linked to therapies involving spinal manipulation, including osteopathy.

These include the tearing of an artery wall leading to a stroke, which can result in permanent disability or even death.

These events usually occurred after spinal manipulation involving the neck.

Your osteopath should explain the benefits and any potential risks associated with having treatment.

When it shouldn't be used

Osteopathic treatment is tailored to the individual patient. It isn't recommended where there's an increased risk of damage to the spine or other bones, ligaments, joints or nerves.

This means people with certain health conditions may not be able to have osteopathy.

These conditions include:

⇨ osteoporosis

⇨ fractures

⇨ acute inflammatory conditions, such as some types of arthritis

⇨ infections

⇨ blood clotting disorders, such as haemophilia

⇨ cancer

⇨ multiple sclerosis (MS).

Osteopathy is also not recommended if you're taking blood-thinning medicines, such as warfarin, are having a course of radiotherapy, or during pregnancy.

Osteopaths are trained to use their clinical judgement to identify patients for whom osteopathic treatment isn't appropriate.

To judge whether a health treatment is safe and effective, we need evidence gathered by conducting fair scientific tests.

What evidence is there?

Most research into techniques used in osteopathy tends to focus on general 'manual therapy' techniques, such as spinal manipulation.

Manual therapy techniques are used by physiotherapists and chiropractors, as well as osteopaths.

The National Institute for Health and Care Excellence (NICE) guidelines on managing lower back pain and sciatica state that manual therapy can be considered as a treatment option alongside exercise.

NICE also recommends manual therapy as a possible treatment option for osteoarthritis, but osteopathy isn't specifically mentioned.

There's only limited or no scientific evidence to support osteopathy as an effective treatment for:

⇨ asthma

⇨ painful periods

⇨ excessive crying in babies (colic)

⇨ glue ear

⇨ problems affecting the jaw (temporomandibular disorder)

⇨ abnormal curvature of the spine (scoliosis)

⇨ placebo effect.

When we use a treatment and feel better, this can sometimes happen because of a phenomenon called the placebo effect and not because of the treatment itself.

This means that, although many people treated by osteopaths report good results, it's not always clear how effective the treatment actually is for certain conditions.

29 May 2018

⇨ The above information is reproduced with kind permission from the NHS. Please visit www. nhs.uk for further information.

What is Chinese herbal medicine?

Chinese herbal medicine is one of the great herbal systems of the world, with an unbroken tradition going back to the 3rd century BC.

Yet throughout its history it has continually developed in response to changing clinical conditions, and has been sustained by research into every aspect of its use. This process continues today with the development of modern medical diagnostic techniques and knowledge.

Because of its systematic approach and clinical effectiveness it has for centuries had a very great influence on the theory and practise of medicine in the East, and more recently has grown rapidly in popularity in the West. It still forms a major part of healthcare provision in China, and is provided in state hospitals alongside western medicine. Chinese medicine includes all oriental traditions emerging from Southeast Asia that have their origins in China.

Practitioners may work within a tradition that comes from Japan, Vietnam, Taiwan or Korea. It is a complete medical system that is capable of treating a very wide range of conditions. It includes herbal therapy, acupuncture, dietary therapy, and exercises in breathing and movement (tai chi and qi gong). Some or several of these may be employed in the course of treatment.

Chinese herbal medicine, along with the other components of Chinese medicine, is based on the concepts of yin and yang. It aims to understand and treat the many ways in which the fundamental balance and harmony between the two may be undermined and the ways in which a person's qi or vitality may be depleted or blocked. Clinical strategies are based upon diagnosis of patterns of signs and symptoms that reflect an imbalance.

However, the tradition as a whole places great emphasis on lifestyle management in order to prevent disease before it occurs. Chinese medicine recognises that health is more than just the absence of disease and it has a unique capacity to maintain and enhance our capacity for well-being and happiness.

What does the Register of Chinese Herbal Medicine (RCHM) believe that Chinese medicine can treat?

The RCHM's Code of Ethics, to which all RCHM members must adhere states that: 'Herbal practitioners must always be aware of the necessity to communicate with other healthcare professionals, directly or indirectly, when the expertise of such professionals fits more properly the needs of a particular patient.'

RCHM members will therefore not discourage essential medical treatment for conditions where western medical supervision or advice should be sought. They will always advise patients, in the case of serious illnesses or uncertain diagnosis, to seek advice and treatment from their GP/consultant. RCHM members will also, with the patient's consent, liaise with that patient's other health professionals, where appropriate, when offering complementary treatment.

The RCHM believes that Chinese herbal medicine has a role to play in the treatment of the following conditions:

⇨ Skin disease, including eczema, psoriasis, acne, rosacea, urticaria

⇨ Gastro-intestinal disorders, including irritable bowel syndrome, chronic constipation, ulcerative colitis

⇨ Gynaecological conditions, including pre-menstrual syndrome and dysmenorrhoea, endometriosis, infertility

- ⇨ Hepatitis and HIV: some promising results have been obtained for treatment of Hepatitis C, and supportive treatment may be beneficial in the case of HIV

- ⇨ Chronic fatigue syndromes, whether with a background of viral infection or in other situations

- ⇨ Respiratory conditions, including asthma, bronchitis, and chronic coughs, allergic and perennial rhinitis and sinusitis

- ⇨ Rheumatological conditions (e.g. osteoarthritis and rheumatoid arthritis)

- ⇨ Urinary conditions including chronic cystitis

- ⇨ Psychological problems (e.g. depression, anxiety).

Many of these conditions, especially in their chronic forms, create great difficulty for conventional medicine, whilst Chinese herbal medicine has a great deal to offer. The results that can be expected and how long a patient will have to take the herbs for will depend on the severity of the condition, its duration, and the general health of the patient.

Any RCHM member will be happy to discuss their experience of treating your type of problem with you before you commit yourself to taking Chinese herbal medicine.

Who can take Chinese herbal medicine?

Chinese medicine can be used by people of any age or constitution. Your practitioner will take any previous or current illness or medication into account before prescribing herbs to you. With suitable adjustments for dosage and with some provisos which will be determined by your practitioner, children and pregnant women can very well be treated by Chinese medicine.

What are the herbs like and how much will they cost?

Herbs are now available in a number of formats, both traditional and modern. The traditional method is to boil a mixture of dried herbs to make a tea or to use pills. The herbs are also now commonly prescribed as freeze-dried powders or tinctures. The herbs will at first taste unusual and often bitter to anyone who has not tried them before, but the vast majority of people get used to the taste very quickly.

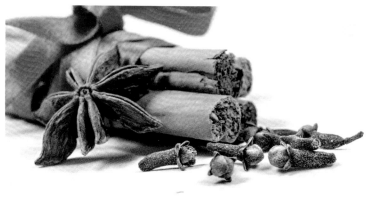

There are no standard prices for consultations or for herbs. This will depend on the individual practitioner and the part of the country you are in. You should enquire about charges when making your appointment.

Many private health insurance companies are now covering acupuncture and a few will also pay for herbal treatment. You should contact your insurance company to check.

Are herbs safe?

Chinese herbs are very safe when prescribed correctly by a properly trained practitioner. Over the centuries doctors have compiled detailed information about the pharmacopoeia and placed great emphasis on the protection of the patient. Adverse reactions can occur with any form of medicine. In the case of Chinese herbal medicine these are rare. RCHM members give guidance on this to all patients.

The RCHM also works with the Bristol Chinese Herb Garden and with the Royal Botanic Gardens, Kew, in building botanical knowledge of high quality herbal medicines.

Endangered species

The RCHM is greatly concerned about the threat to wild animals and plants that have come as a result of the growth in demand for traditional medicines. We strongly condemn the illegal trade in endangered species and have a strict policy prohibiting the use of any type of endangered species by any of our Members.

The RCHM uses information supplied by the Convention on International Trade in Endangered Species (CITES), the Wildlife Liaison Office of the Metropolitan Police and the Department of the Environment, all of whom work to stop the trade in illegal substances wherever it is found.

Herbal medicine and modern pharmacology

There is a growing body of research which indicates that traditional uses of plant remedies and the known pharmacological activity of plant constituents often coincide. However, herbal medicine is distinct from medicine based on pharmaceutical drugs. Firstly, because of the complexity of plant materials it is far more balanced than medicine based on isolated active ingredients and is far less likely to cause side effects. Secondly, because herbs are typically prescribed in combination, the different components of a formulae balance each other, and they undergo a mutual synergy which increases efficacy and enhances safety. Thirdly, herbal medicine seeks primarily to correct internal imbalances rather than to treat symptoms alone, and therapeutic intervention is designed to encourage this self-healing process.

- ⇨ The above information is reprinted with kind permission from the RCHM. Please visit www.rchm.co.uk for further information.

© 2018 Register of Chinese Herbal Medicine

Complementary therapies

Read about different types of complementary therapy that some people find helpful.

Acupuncture

Western medical acupuncture is based on current medical knowledge and evidence-based medicine. It is very similar to traditional acupuncture. This technique involves inserting sterile needles into certain 'trigger points' just below the skin. This is thought to stimulate the nerves and cause the release of natural chemicals into the body, which may give you a feeling of well-being. It is advised that you avoid acupuncture if you have low immunity or lymphoedema. Acupuncture is a physical therapy.

Aromatherapy

The use of natural oils extracted from plants is called aromatherapy. They are used during massage, in baths and creams or through diffusers. Many people find aromatherapy a relaxing and enjoyable experience. Aromatherapy is part of a group of therapies that use herb and plant extracts.

Art therapy

Art therapy helps you to express feelings by painting, drawing or sculpting. Being creative can sometimes help you become more aware of, and let go of, difficult feelings. Feelings can then be discussed in groups or counselling. Art therapy is a mind-body therapy. It is not widely available in the NHS.

Counselling

If you need to talk to someone outside your circle of family and friends, you may find speaking to a counsellor or psychologist can help. Counsellors and psychologists are trained to listen. They can help you explore your feelings and talk through confusing or upsetting emotions. Counselling is a psychological therapy.

Diet and food supplements

In general, cancer experts recommend following a healthy, balanced diet. People often ask their doctor about special diets but there isn't enough clear information to make exact recommendations about what someone with cancer should eat. Each person's needs are different. A dietitian can give you advice on what to eat and may prescribe supplements if you need them.

Flower remedies

Flower remedies come from the essence of flowers diluted many times. People who use flower remedies feel they help reduce anxiety and help them feel better. Flower remedies are part of a group of therapies that use herb and plant extracts.

Herbal remedies

Herbal remedies may be drunk as a tea or taken as a tablet, cream or ointment. Some herbs can interact with conventional treatment, so it is important to speak to your doctor before taking them. Herbal therapy is part of a group of therapies that use herb and plant extracts.

Homeopathy

Homeopathy may be used with conventional treatment to try to improve the quality of life for people with cancer. There is no reliable medical evidence that homeopathy is effective. It involves taking a remedy that causes similar symptoms to the illness being treated. By doing this, therapists aim to trigger the body's natural reaction. Some GPs and hospital doctors are trained in homeopathy, and it is sometimes available through the NHS. Homeopathy is part of a group of therapies that use herb and plant extracts.

Hypnotherapy

Hypnotherapy may help you to make positive lifestyle changes or to encourage positive emotions, such as calmness and relaxation. Hypnotherapists work with you to create a helpful state of mind. The therapist will make suggestions, which are believed to have a helpful effect on the way you deal with certain situations. Hypnotherapy is a mind-body therapy.

Massage therapy

Massage is a form of structured or therapeutic touch. There are many types of massage. Some are soft and gentle, while others are more active. Massage therapy can be used to relax your mind and body, relieve tension and may enhance your mood. Massage therapists working with people with cancer must be properly trained and qualified.

Meditation

Meditation uses concentration or reflection to deeply relax and calm the mind. This can help reduce feelings of fear, pain, anxiety and depression. Regular meditation practice can help people feel more in control of themselves and their lives. Meditation is a mind-body therapy.

Mindfulness meditation

Mindfulness meditation is an approach that can help you change the way you think about different experiences. Therapists help you to pay attention to the present moment and to be aware of your thoughts and feelings. Using mediation, breathing and yoga, therapists aim to encourage positive thought and to break cycles of negative thought and behaviour. This is a psychological therapy.

Music therapy

This therapy uses music to improve quality of life, by helping people communicate. You don't need to be able to play an instrument or read music. During the session, you work with a range of easy-to-use instruments. Music therapy is a mind-body therapy. It is not widely available in the NHS.

Reflexology

By applying gentle pressure to specific points on the hands or feet, reflexology aims to help you relax. Reflexologists believe different areas on hands or feet represent, and are connected to, different parts of the body. Reflexology is an energy-based therapy.

Relaxation

Relaxation therapy aims to reduce anxiety and stress by using simple breathing and relaxation exercises. There are different relaxation techniques you can use at home or as part of a group. Relaxation is a mind-body therapy.

Self-help groups

Joining a group of people affected by cancer gives you a chance to share experiences. If you need help dealing with certain emotions, self-help groups can offer different techniques and coping strategies. They can also be a great source of practical information and emotional support. Self-help groups are a type of psychological therapy.

Shiatsu and acupressure

Shiatsu is a Japanese form of massage. Acupressure is similar as therapists use their hands or elbows to apply pressure to certain areas of the body. Therapists believe that health depends

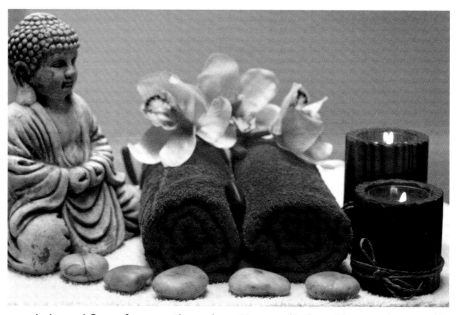

on a balanced flow of energy through certain channels in the body. Their theory is that placing pressure on these channels helps restore energy balance. Shiatsu and acupressure are energy-based therapies.

Support groups

This is when a trained therapist (counsellor or other professional) encourages a group of people to share their feelings and experiences with each other. The therapist is aware of each individual's problems and guides the session to ensure everyone benefits. Support or group therapy is a psychological therapy.

Tai chi and qi gong

These therapies use gentle, controlled, low-impact movements combined with breathing exercises. They bring physical and mental exercises together to improve your health and to create a feeling of well-being. They form part of a group of physical therapies.

Therapeutic touch

In therapeutic touch, the therapist uses touch or works just above the surface of the body. They believe this affects an energy field surrounding each person and they can act as a channel for the healing energy. Reiki is a type of therapeutic touch.

No medical evidence shows this helps with symptoms or side effects, but many people feel that this therapy gives them valuable support. Therapeutic touch is an energy-based therapy.

Visualisation

This therapy involves creating images in your mind while in a state of relaxation or meditation. The theory is that by imagining a peaceful scene, you will feel more relaxed. Visualisation is a mind-body therapy.

Yoga

Yoga involves positioning your body in different ways and doing breathing exercises. There are different types, and most use some form of meditation or relaxation. Some use very gentle stretches, movement and meditation. Others involve more vigorous physical movements and dietary changes. Yoga is part of a group of physical therapies.

⇨ The above information is reprinted with kind permission from Macmillan Cancer Support. Please visit www.macmillan.org.uk for further information.

Traditional African medicine and conventional drugs: friends or enemies?

An article from **The Conversation.**

THE CONVERSATION

By Chrisna Gouws, Senior Lecturer, North-West University

Africa is home to an extensive and diverse medicinal plant life. This includes commonly used herbs like Rooibos (*Aspalathus linearis*), Devil's claw (*Harpagophytum procumbens*), Buchu (*Agathosma betulina*), Cape Aloe (*Aloe ferox*) and Hoodia (*Hoodia gordonii*).

These plant – or herb-based treatments have been a key part of the continent's traditional medicinal practices for thousands of years. Up to 80% of people in some areas regularly use traditional medicines and consult traditional health practitioners. In some areas, traditional treatments are the main or only treatment because they are accessible, affordable and culturally accepted.

Numerous traditional African medicines are undeniably beneficial in treating disease or maintaining good health. Some have even been the source of many prescription medicines. But there are challenges. These include the fact that many consumers automatically assume 'natural equals safe'. Another problem arises when people use traditional or herbal remedies together with prescribed medicines.

Part of the research my colleagues and I do at North-West University in South Africa is focused on understanding these combinations. Which are harmful? Which could be beneficial? We're looking at what's known as 'interactions' – the effect herbal medicines may have on the normal uptake, breakdown or activity of prescribed medicines.

Knowledge is key. Scientists need to conduct proper research to understand such interactions. Consumers need to be taught about these interactions, whether good or bad, and to tell their healthcare providers about everything they're taking.

Understanding interactions

Prescriptions of traditional African medicines tend to be secretive. They're based on knowledge passed from generation to generation of traditional healers. This can result in vague doses. Patients have been known to overuse some remedies while self-medicating. This can have severe health consequences. These include stomach upsets, liver damage and even kidney failure. Some widely used natural health plant products which have been associated with adverse health effects because of

misuse include *Aloe vera*, Echinacea (*Echinacea purpurea*) and Green tea (*Camellia sinensis*).

All of these natural remedies are generally considered 'safe', or even healthy by consumers since their use is not regulated or restricted. Nothing indicates to the user that 'too much of a good thing' could be dangerous.

Thanks partly to efforts by the World Health Organization, access to Western medicine – especially for diseases like HIV/AIDS – is increasing across Africa. More and more people tend to be using traditional medicine in combination with prescription medicines. Often none of their healthcare providers know about this and so cannot warn about possible interactions.

Some traditional African medicines may interfere with the normal metabolism of drugs. For example, St John's wort is a natural remedy frequently used for depression. But it's been shown to increase the removal of medicines, such as some oral contraceptives, from the body. This can lead to ineffective levels of the prescribed medicine, putting women at risk of pregnancy when they think they are protected.

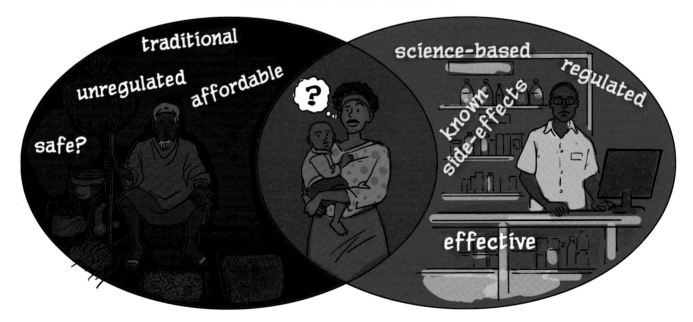

On the other hand, the interaction could also result in reduced clearance of a drug. This may lead to higher levels of the prescribed medicine in the body, which produces negative side effects and could even lead to toxicity.

These interactions happen at a metabolic level. So even herbal products that are safe when used on their own may pose a risk when taken in combination with Western medicine – that is, synthetic pharmaceutical agents.

Some of the best known examples of drug interactions are the effects of citrus, particularly grapefruit juice, and alcohol of many prescribed medicines. These combinations should be avoided.

Another example of particular importance in Africa is Cancer bush (*Sutherlandia frutescens*). It is widely used in the treatment of diseases such as HIV/AIDS and TB, especially in countries like Zambia, Swaziland, Zimbabwe and South Africa, as it is believed to generally improve quality of life in these patients. But it has been shown to lower the plasma levels of the antiretroviral drug, atazanavir, to sub-therapeutic levels when they're taken together, reducing its anti-HIV efficacy.

This traditional remedy can also interfere with isoniazid therapy, which is used as a preventative measure in TB treatment.

Despite these known interactions, policy makers still promote the use of these herbal remedies in the management of HIV/AIDS and associated illnesses. Clearly more public engagement is needed so patients understand the risks of interaction.

And the good news

But it's not all bad news. Interactions between African traditional medicines and prescribed medicines can potentially be exploited for good.

One of the biggest problems in the development of new medicines is the low uptake of these compounds into the body, or its quick removal. In some studies, traditional medicines have been shown to have the ability to increase uptake or decrease the metabolism of prescription drugs. Applying these effects could enable the development of new herb-drug combinations with increased efficacy and reduced side effects.

But studies that characterise and evaluate the healing properties or potential toxicity and drug interactions of traditional African medicines are very limited. This is further complicated by the fact that so many medicinal plants (more than 5,000) are being used. So healthcare practitioners have limited information and often can't make proper recommendations to patients who use such traditional remedies.

Whether positive or negative drug interactions are at play, African countries need to improve their regulation around traditional medicines. Only a few, among them Nigeria, Cameroon and South Africa, have incorporated traditional African medicines into their adverse drug reaction reporting systems.

5 March 2018

⇨ The above information is reprinted with kind permission from *The Conversation*. Please visit www.theconversation.com for further information.

Homeopathy

Homeopathy is a 'treatment' based on the use of highly diluted substances, which practitioners claim can cause the body to heal itself.

A 2010 House of Commons Science and Technology Committee report on homeopathy said that homeopathic remedies perform no better than placebos (dummy treatments).

The review also said that the principles on which homeopathy is based are 'scientifically implausible'.

This is also the view of the Chief Medical Officer, Professor Dame Sally Davies.

What is homeopathy?

Homeopathy is a complementary or alternative medicine (CAM). This means that homeopathy is different from treatments that are part of conventional Western medicine in important ways.

It's based on a series of ideas developed in the 1790s by a German doctor called Samuel Hahnemann.

A central principle of the 'treatment' is that 'like cures like' – that a substance that causes certain symptoms can also help to remove those symptoms.

A second central principle is based around a process of dilution and shaking called succussion.

Practitioners believe that the more a substance is diluted in this way, the greater its power to treat symptoms.

Many homeopathic remedies consist of substances that have been diluted many times in water until there's none, or almost none, of the original substance left.

Homeopathy is used to 'treat' an extremely wide range of conditions, including physical conditions such as asthma and psychological conditions such as depression.

Does it work?

There's been extensive investigation of the effectiveness of homeopathy. There's no good-quality evidence that homeopathy is effective as a treatment for any health condition.

Is it available on the NHS?

Homeopathy isn't widely available on the NHS. In 2017, NHS England recommended that GPs and other prescribers should stop providing it.

This is because they found no clear or robust evidence to support the use of homeopathy on the NHS.

Homeopathy is usually practised privately, and homeopathic remedies are available from pharmacies.

The price for a consultation with a homeopath can vary from around £30 to £125. Homeopathic tablets or other products usually cost around £4 to £10.

What should I expect if I try it?

When you first see a homeopath, they'll usually ask you about any specific health conditions, but also ask about your general well-being, emotional state, lifestyle and diet.

Based on this, the homeopath will decide on the course of treatment, which most often takes the form of homeopathic remedies given as a pill, capsule or tincture (solution).

Your homeopath may recommend that you attend one or more follow-up appointments so the remedy's effects on your health can be assessed.

When is it used?

Homeopathy is used for an extremely wide range of health conditions. Many practitioners believe it can help with any condition.

Among the most common conditions that people seek homeopathic treatment for are:

⇨ asthma

⇨ ear infections

⇨ hay fever

⇨ mental health conditions, such as depression, stress and anxiety

⇨ allergies, such as food allergies

⇨ dermatitis (an allergic skin condition)

⇨ arthritis

⇨ high blood pressure.

There's no good-quality evidence that homeopathy is an effective treatment for these or any other health conditions.

Some practitioners also claim homeopathy can prevent malaria or other diseases. There's no evidence to support this, and no scientifically plausible way that homeopathy can prevent diseases.

The National Institute for Health and Care Excellence (NICE) advises the NHS on the proper use of treatments.

Currently, NICE doesn't recommend that homeopathy should be used in the treatment of any health condition.

What are the regulation issues?

There's no legal regulation of homeopathic practitioners in the UK. This means that anyone can practise as a homeopath, even if they have no qualifications or experience.

Voluntary regulation aims to protect patient safety, but it doesn't mean there's scientific evidence that a treatment is effective.

A number of professional associations can help you find a homeopath who will practise the treatment in a way that's acceptable to you.

The Society of Homeopaths and the Federation of Holistic Therapists both have a register of homeopathy practitioners, which you can search to find a practitioner near you. These registers are accredited by the Professional Standards Authority.

Is it safe?

Homeopathic remedies are generally safe, and the risk of a serious adverse side effect arising from taking these remedies is thought to be small.

Some homeopathic remedies may contain substances that aren't safe or interfere with the action of other medicines.

You should talk to your GP before stopping any treatment prescribed by a doctor, or avoiding procedures such as vaccination, in favour of homeopathy.

What can we conclude from the evidence?

There have been several reviews of the scientific evidence on the effectiveness of homeopathy.

The House of Commons Science and Technology Committee said there's

no evidence that homeopathy is effective as a treatment for any health condition.

There's no evidence behind the idea that substances that cause certain symptoms can also help treat them.

Nor is there any evidence behind the idea that diluting and shaking substances in water can turn those substances into medicines.

The ideas that underpin homeopathy aren't accepted by mainstream science, and aren't consistent with long-accepted principles on the way the physical world works.

The Committee's 2010 report on homeopathy said the 'like cures like' principle is 'theoretically weak', and that this is the 'settled view of medical science'.

For example, many homeopathic remedies are diluted to such an extent that it's unlikely there's a single molecule of the original substance remaining in the final remedy. In cases like these, homeopathic remedies consist of nothing but water.

Some homeopaths believe that, as a result of the succussion process, the original substance leaves an 'imprint' of itself on the water. But there's no known mechanism by which this can occur.

The 2010 report said: 'We consider the notion that ultra-dilutions can maintain an imprint of substances previously dissolved in them to be scientifically implausible.'

Some people who use homeopathy may see an improvement in their health condition as the result of a phenomenon known as the placebo effect.

If you choose health treatments that provide only a placebo effect, you may miss out on other treatments that have been proven to be more effective.

23 March 2018

⇨ The above information is reproduced with kind permission from the NHS. Please visit www.nhs.uk for further information.

Alexander Technique

Alexander Technique teaches improved posture and movement, which is believed to help reduce and prevent problems caused by unhelpful habits.

During a number of lessons you're taught to be more aware of your body, how to improve poor posture and move more efficiently.

Teachers of the Alexander Technique believe it helps get rid of tension in your body and relieves problems such as back pain, neck ache, sore shoulders and other musculoskeletal problems.

Evidence suggests the technique has the potential to improve certain health conditions, but there are some claims made about the technique that haven't been scientifically tested.

Key principles

The main principles of the Alexander Technique are:

⇨ 'how you move, sit and stand affects how well you function'

⇨ 'the relationship of the head, neck and spine is fundamental to your ability to function optimally'

⇨ 'becoming more mindful of the way you go about your daily activities is necessary to make changes and gain benefit'

⇨ 'the mind and body work together intimately as one, each constantly influencing the other'.

Teachers of the technique say that conditions such as backache and other sorts of long-term pain are often the result of misusing your body over a long period of time, such as moving inefficiently and standing or sitting with your weight unevenly distributed.

The aim of the Alexander Technique is to help you 'unlearn' these bad habits and achieve a balanced, more naturally aligned body.

Learning the Alexander Technique

The Alexander Technique is taught by a qualified teacher in one-to-one lessons.

Lessons often take place in a studio, clinic or the teacher's house and usually last 30 to 45 minutes. You'll be asked to wear loose-fitting, comfortable clothing so you're able to move easily.

The teacher will observe your movements and show you how to move, sit, lie down and stand with better balance and less strain. They'll use their hands to gently guide you in your movements, help you maintain a better relationship between your head, neck and spine, and to release muscle tension.

You'll need to attend a number of lessons to learn the basic concepts of the Alexander Technique. Often, around 20 or more weekly lessons are recommended.

Teachers of the technique say you may see an improvement in aches and pains fairly soon after starting the lessons, but that you need to be committed to putting what you learn into practice and it may take a considerable amount of time to see the full benefits.

The overall aim is to help you gain an understanding of the main principles involved so you can apply them to everyday life, allowing you to benefit from the technique without the need for frequent ongoing lessons.

Does it work?

Proponents of the Alexander Technique often claim it can help people with a wide range of health conditions. Some of these claims are supported by scientific evidence, but some have not yet been properly tested.

There's evidence suggesting the Alexander Technique can help people with:

⇨ **long-term back pain** – lessons in the technique may lead to reduced back pain-associated disability and reduce how often you feel pain for up to a year or more

⇨ **long-term neck pain** – lessons in the technique may lead to reduced neck pain and associated disability for up to a year or more

⇨ **Parkinson's disease** – lessons in the technique may help you carry out everyday tasks more easily and improve how you feel about your condition.

If you have one of these conditions and are considering trying the Alexander Technique, it's a good idea to speak to your GP or specialist first to check if it might be suitable for you.

Some research has also suggested the Alexander Technique may improve general long-term pain, stammering and balance skills in elderly people to help them avoid falls. But the evidence in these areas is limited and more studies are needed.

There's currently little evidence to suggest the Alexander Technique can help improve other health conditions, including asthma, headaches, osteoarthritis, difficulty sleeping (insomnia) and stress.

8 June 2018

⇨ The above information is an extract from the article *Alexander technique* and is reproduced with kind permission from the NHS. Please visit www.nhs.uk for further information.

Reiki

Reiki, pronounced 'ray-key', is a system of energy healing originating from Japan. The word reiki itself translates to 'universal life energy' and is based on the belief that life energy flows through all living things. When this energy becomes disrupted or blocked, it is believed that stress and disease follow.

Reiki practitioners use the universal life energy they have been attuned to, to promote natural healing. In this article we will explore reiki healing in more depth to establish what it can help with and what you should expect from a reiki session.

What is Reiki?

In a similar vein to many traditional eastern therapies, reiki works on the premise that 'life force energy' flows through all of us. If this energy becomes unbalanced, low or stuck, it is believed that we are more likely to become stressed and unwell.

Reiki is carried out by practitioners who have been attuned to the reiki energy. This attunement involves a reiki master who acts as a mirror to help the student adjust to the energy. This creates a channel between the practitioner and the universal life energy so they can access and use the energy to help others.

Using their hands, reiki practitioners use this energy to help balance clients' energy. The nature of reiki is holistic, meaning that it addresses the body, mind and spirit. While reiki is considered spiritual, it is not a religion. There is nothing specific you need to believe in, in order to benefit from reiki healing.

This method of energy healing promotes relaxation and well-being. Its aim is to help reduce stress and stimulate the body's natural healing abilities. Mikao Usui founded the practice in the early 20th century.

Dr Usui described the five principles of reiki for practitioners to consider, which are:

1. Just for today, do not worry.

2. Just for today, do not anger.

3. Honour your parents, teachers and elders.

4. Earn your living honestly.

5. Show gratitude for every living thing.

'As running water smoothes the jagged edges of a rock until it is small enough to roll away, reiki flows to the areas of need, soothing and supporting the body's natural ability to heal itself.'

Energy healing

Any treatment that works with energy typically falls under the energy healing umbrella. Each provides similar rebalancing and relaxation benefits. Having said this, there are differences in the theoretical foundations and how practitioners are trained.

Energy healing tends to use touch techniques that require healing powers from the therapists themselves. Therapists will then channel energy into the recipient to bring about healing. Energy healers (sometimes referred to as spiritual healers) may believe they are more vulnerable to other entities, picking up negative energy from the person they are working on. They therefore need to carry out steps to protect themselves. Reiki healers are believed to be protected by the attunement process.

What can reiki help with?

The relaxing nature of reiki makes it beneficial in many situations. It can be especially helpful for those who may be feeling disconnected, isolated or overwhelmed. Reiki can help to bring about a sense of peace and centredness, helping you feel better able to cope with challenges.

The calming effect of a reiki treatment is also beneficial to pregnant women, supporting them on their journey. Children and even animals can benefit from reiki as it relaxes and soothes.

Promoting a sense of well-being, many find reiki encourages and supports positive lifestyle choices. Some even say it helps to reduce the need for alcohol and tobacco.

When used in conjunction with medical treatment, rebalancing energy can help to manage symptoms of anxiety, fatigue and pain. Reiki can be used for short-term problems or in an ongoing capacity to promote overall health and well-being.

Remember, reiki is a complementary therapy. If you have a health concern, visit your doctor and seek medical advice. Reiki should not be used in place of your doctor's recommendations; it should be used alongside your treatment to aid healing. Because reiki is a natural treatment there are no contraindications, meaning it is generally safe to use for everyone. You are advised, however, to discuss your medical history with your reiki practitioner in case they need to take extra precautions.

A typical session

Before you begin your treatment, your reiki practitioner will explain to you what the treatment involves. During this consultation, they may ask you why you are seeking reiki and details of your medical history. Providing as much detail as possible here ensures that they treat you safely and to the best of their ability.

After this consultation you will be asked to sit or lie down in a comfortable position. You do not need to remove your clothing for reiki healing. For comfort you may wish to remove constricting layers, shoes and/ or glasses.

The treatment itself involves the practitioner placing their hands gently on the body, or slightly above the body, in a predetermined sequence. The position of the hands is non-intrusive and should not cause any discomfort. If you feel uncomfortable at any point, let your therapist know. The amount of time spent in each position will depend on the nature of your concern. The touch should be gentle and light, reiki is not supposed to manipulate or massage.

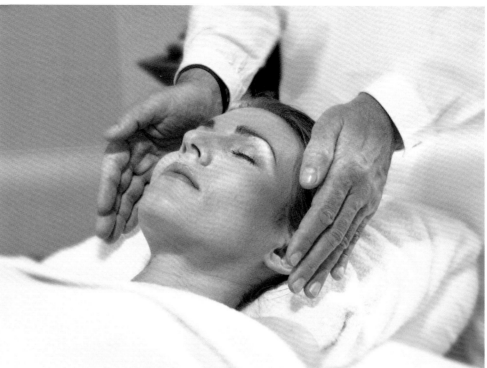

How will I feel?

Everyone will respond differently to reiki depending on their individual circumstances. Some people say they feel sensations during their reiki healing, while others do not. Some feel heat or tingling during the treatment and some report seeing colours. For some, the experience brings up an emotional response. The most common response, however, is a feeling of calm, relaxation and well-being.

After the treatment you may feel very relaxed, or you may feel energised. There is no right or wrong way to experience reiki. Some people say after the treatment they encounter a 'healing reaction', like a headache or flu-like symptoms. If you are concerned about any reaction, speak to your practitioner.

How many sessions will I need?

This will vary from person to person. It is important to remember that reiki healing is a process, and therefore may take a number of sessions. Generally, the more chronic and long term the concern is, the more sessions it will require.

Your practitioner may recommend a number and/or the spacing of your sessions. You should, however, feel free to make the decision about the spacing of your treatment yourself.

How do I choose a practitioner?

Reiki is not a regulated therapy, which means there are no laws in place surrounding practitioners. Reiki practitioners should have undergone certain levels of training before they practise on clients – these are described below:

Level 1 (first degree): This is an introductory level that opens up energy channels on a physical level. This allows practitioners to connect to the universal life force energy. The goal of level 1 reiki training is to practise self-healing.

Level 2 (second degree): Once this level has been completed, practitioners receive the 'Reiki Symbols'. These allow the practitioner to connect more deeply with the universal energy. This in turn allows them to use reiki on other people.

Level 3 (third degree/Reiki Master): This is considered a teacher's level and is not required before treating clients. Graduates are able to 'attune' new Reiki practitioners after completing level 3. Becoming a Reiki Master signifies a deep commitment to the reiki practice.

When it comes to picking a practitioner, it's important to check they have level 2 training (or equivalent) so they can practise on other people. On Therapy Directory, all members are checked to ensure they meet this criteria.

Once you have established the level of training, finding out more about the practitioner can help you decide. Find out more about their journey with reiki and if possible, read some testimonials. On Therapy Directory we encourage all members to fill their profiles with information so you can find out more about them before booking a session.

Ultimately, you will want to book an appointment with someone who you feel comfortable with, so you can truly relax during the treatment. Follow your intuition and feel free to call or email them to find out more about the way they work.

⇨ The above information is reprinted with kind permission from Therapy Directory. Please visit www.therapy-directory.org.uk for further information.

© 2018 Therapy Directory

What is herbal medicine?

What is a herbalist?

A herbalist is a healthcare professional who uses plants or plant extracts to treat health conditions and to improve health and well-being. Medical herbalists make use of plants whose traditional uses are backed up by modern scientific research and clinical trials. A qualified medical herbalist has a BSc or equivalent in Herbal Medicine, has studied orthodox medicine as well as plant medicine and is trained in the same diagnostic skills as a GP. However, herbalists take an holistic approach to illness, treating the underlying cause of disease rather than just the symptoms. They are able to prescribe herbal remedies to be used alongside other medication and treatments, and many patients are referred to a herbalist by their GP for treatment.

Herbal medicine is suitable for people of any age, including children, who respond especially well to the gentle actions of herbs. Each patient is treated as an individual – a medical herbalist recognises that no two patients are the same.

What is herbal medicine?

Herbal medicines are plant-based medicines made from differing combinations of plant parts, e.g. leaves, flowers or roots. Each part can have different medicinal uses and the many types of chemical constituents require different extraction methods. Both fresh and dried plant matter are used, depending on the herb.

The National Institute of Medical Herbalists members are aware of the importance of medicines being sourced from reputable manufacturers, who maintain consistent quality standards. Traceability (right back to the original batch of herbs) and certificates of authenticity are key ways in which quality is maintained. Sustainability is also of crucial importance.

Water-based preparations
⇨ Infusions: dried or fresh herbs, usually aerial parts, steeped in boiling water

⇨ Decoction: usually harder plant material, boiled on the stove for longer than infusions

⇨ Syrups: herbs incorporated into a thick, sweet liquid

⇨ Poultices: moistened herbs kept in place by a cloth for localised healing

⇨ Lotions: infusions or decoctions delivered in a smooth liquid preparation

⇨ Compresses: generally a soft cloth wrung out of a hot or cold infusion or decoction and applied to the affected area

Alcohol-based preparations, usually called tinctures. There are non-alcoholic alternatives to this such as glycerites or vinegars, which are taken in the same way.

Oil-based preparations such as infused oils and ointments are used externally.

Other preparations commonly used:

⇨ Powders taken internally and applied externally, may come in loose form or in capsules

⇨ Juices are very nutritive

⇨ Creams are often preferred in the treatment of skin conditions

⇨ Steam inhalations

⇨ Baths and skin washes

⇨ Gargles and mouthwashes

⇨ Pessaries and suppositories.

What does a herbalist treat?

Medical herbalism is for everyone – if you would like more specific information on how a medical herbalist approaches health problems, please see categories below on our website or contact your local medical herbalist.

⇨ Joints and Bone

⇨ Heart and Circulation

⇨ Skin

⇨ Nutrition and Nourishment

⇨ Fertility, Pregnancy and Childbirth

⇨ Hormone Health

⇨ Emotional Health

⇨ Fatigue Syndrome

⇨ Energy and Stamina

⇨ Digestion

⇨ Allergy

⇨ The Immune System

What happens during a consultation?

During your first consultation with a medical herbalist, the medical herbalist will build up a picture of you and your health by:

⇨ Taking your full case history

⇨ Asking about your family's medical history

⇨ Discussing your diet and lifestyle

⇨ Finding out about any medication or supplements you use.

This allows your herbalist to assess the underlying causes of your illness and formulate a mixture of herbs tailored to your individual needs. It may also be necessary to take your blood pressure or arrange for other tests to be done.

Your individual treatment plan will include herbal remedies and, where appropriate, dietary changes or nutritional supplements. Most herbal medicines are given in the form of a liquid tincture that is taken in 5ml doses of two or three times daily. You may also be prescribed a herbal tea, tablets, ointment, cream or lotion.

After the initial consultation, three or four shorter consultations are usually necessary to assess your progress, followed by check-ups every three to six months, depending on the nature of your condition. Because herbal medicines work in a gentle and subtle way, they can take longer to work than orthodox drugs, but their effects are long lasting and there should be no side effects.

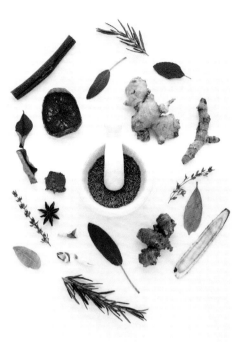

Can herbal medicine be used as first aid?

Medicinal plants have always been used as natural first-aid remedies such as rubbing dock leaves onto nettle stings or applying lavender oil to treat burns. You may also come across herbalists running first-aid stations at outdoor festivals. The teams are qualified in advanced first-aid; some are even experienced nurses and paramedics. Herbs are used to treat a vast arrayof acute conditions, in both emergency and non-emergency situations, from insect bites to headaches to serious wounds.

Whilst much of this tradition has been lost in modern times, there is a resurgence of public interest in the use of local plants for minor ailments. Many herbalists run beginners' courses where you can learn more; from plant identification to making remedies.

Can herbs and pharmaceutical drugs be used together?

There are many instances in which herbs and pharmaceutical drugs work well together.

However, in some situations, there can be negative interactions. Some herbs, like St John's wort, cannot be taken along with certain other medicines. Your medical herbalist is trained to know which herbs to use safely and will be able to advise on any situation.

How long will herbal treatment take?

There is no definitive answer because so many variables will influence the duration of treatment. Our biological makeup is as unique as our medical histories and bodies heal at differing rates.

Influential factors affecting length of therapy required include:

⇨ The condition

⇨ Severity of the condition

⇨ How long it has been present

⇨ Past medical history

⇨ Drug history

⇨ Current health status.

Your herbalist may be able to give you an estimated guideline once they have taken a detailed case history. It is important that progress is closely monitored and herbal prescriptions are adjusted accordingly over time.

Herbal medicines can sometimes take longer before beginning to achieve their desired effect when compared to pharmaceutical drugs. However, their gentle, supportive action aims to address the root cause of the condition and therefore usually produces more permanent results. In addition, when correctly prescribed, side effects are rare.

Whilst the above is applicable for chronic cases, the right dose of herbs can produce immediate results. Medical herbalists working in first-aid situations often resolve acute issues within hours or days.

As the choice of herbs and appropriate administration are key to safety and efficacy, professional advice is recommended.

Should I tell my GP and specialists that I'm taking herbs?

Yes, most definitely.

We advocate the integrated safe use of medicinal plants for our patients by working with other healthcare practitioners such as GPs, nurse practitioners, and specialists. It is very important that all healthcare providers responsible for your care are fully informed about the herbs and drugs you are taking, including over the counter products and food supplements. This is important in order to avoid possible herb/drug/supplement/food interactions. Your medical herbalist is aware of the difficulties involved and will provide information on request and with your permission will liaise with any of your other healthcare providers.

Medical herbalists often work alongside, and in co-operation with, a wide range of practitioners, including conventional healthcare professionals, and this is something that we are keen to continue and develop.

What happens during a consultation with a medical herbalist?

The first appointment with your medical herbalist will find out about your current health complaint, take a detailed medical history and perform any necessary diagnostic examinations before suggesting a treatment. The consultation will include a full discussion on all aspects of health. It is helpful if the patient can bring to a consultation any information relating to their condition, including information about any pharmaceutical drugs or food supplements that they may be taking.

At the end of the consultation, a tailor-made healthcare plan will be drawn up. This can include herbal medicines (in alcoholic tincture, tea, capsule or cream form), nutritional supplements, diet and lifestyle recommendations. After this there may be a need for a follow-up consultation, to check on progress and to make any necessary adjustments to the healthcare plan.

2017

⇨ The above information is reprinted with kind permission from The National Institute of Medical Herbalists. Please visit www.nimh.org.uk for further information.

Pains and needles: brain scans point to hidden effects of acupuncture

Placebo acupuncture can ease short-term pain but the real thing might help to reverse the underlying pathology of a disease.

By Jo Marchant

Doctors in China have been pushing needles into patients' skin, supposedly to restore the flow of healing 'qi energy', for more than 4,000 years. Sometimes it feels as though researchers in the West have been arguing about the practice for almost as long. After more than 3,000 clinical trials of acupuncture, many scientists are convinced that despite the benefits that patients might think they experience, the whole thing is simply a highly convincing placebo.

But are the sceptics missing something? A steady trickle of neuroscience studies suggests that relying on patients' pain ratings in acupuncture trials might be hiding important changes in the brain.

Just as they do with drugs, scientists test whether acupuncture works against a placebo – a convincing but sham alternative. Methods vary but this often involves placing needles at non-acupuncture points, and using retractable needles that don't penetrate the skin. The aim is to control for the effects of patients' positive belief in a therapy: simply thinking that your pain is about to decline can trigger the brain to release natural pain-relieving molecules called endorphins (a type of opioid, chemically similar to painkillers such as morphine). The central assumption is that such effects occur equally whether patients get a placebo or an actual treatment.

The key test, then, is the difference between the two: if both groups report the same level of pain relief, scientists conclude that the treatment being tested doesn't work. When acupuncture is subjected to trials like this, there is only a small effect above placebo, and often no difference at all.

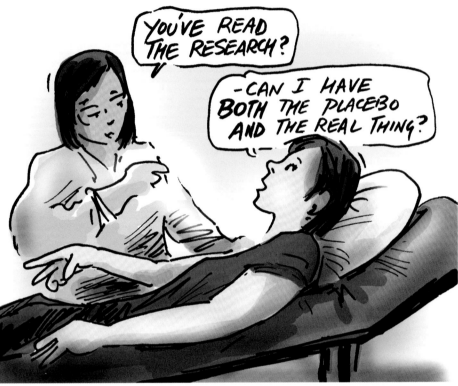

Neuroscientists have been studying how acupuncture affects the brain. It's clear from many imaging studies that causing pain by inserting needles into the skin does influence brain activity, presumably by activating nerves close to the acupuncture point. Intriguingly, being pricked with needles seems to reduce activity in areas of the brain normally associated with pain, dubbed 'the pain matrix', says Hugh MacPherson, an acupuncture researcher at the University of York. 'Rather than activating the pain matrix, it actually de-activates it.'

Sceptics argue that because of the lack of effect in clinical trials, such results are irrelevant. 'It wouldn't be at all surprising if being impaled with needles produced a signal in the brain,' says David Colquhoun, a pharmacologist at University College London and a prominent sceptic of alternative medicine. 'It doesn't tell you anything about how useful the needles are to patients.'

But a new generation of brain imaging studies is suggesting that perhaps researchers should refine their testing methods. There are now several trials showing that even when patients in acupuncture and placebo groups report similar drops in pain, the physical effects of treatment can be very different.

For example, Richard Harris, a neuroscientist at the University of Michigan, Ann Arbor, and colleagues used brain scans to investigate whether acupuncture triggers an endorphin hit in the same way that placebos do. They gave fibromyalgia patients – a condition characterised by chronic, widespread pain – either real or placebo acupuncture (using retractable needles at non-acupuncture points) then scanned their brains using positron emission tomography (PET) imaging. PET scans can't see endorphins directly, but can detect the opioid receptors that these molecules target. Opioid receptors are present on the surface of nerve cells in the brain. When 'locked' by endorphins (or other opioid molecules such as morphine), they prevent the cell from sending pain signals. In Harris' experiment, a drop in the number of free, or unlocked, receptors in the patients' brains would show that endorphins had been released.

After a single acupuncture session, as well as over a month-long course of treatment, both groups of patients reported a similar reduction in pain. In the placebo group, the PET scans did indeed show fewer free opioid receptors in areas of the brain associated with the regulation of pain, suggesting their pain relief was caused by endorphins. Harris assumed that in the real acupuncture group, he'd see something similar. 'I expected that we would probably see the exact same thing between real and sham acupuncture, or that acupuncture might do it better,' he says. Instead, he saw the opposite. Within 45 minutes of the needling session, the number of free opioid receptors in the patients' brains didn't fall; it surged. 'I was completely floored,' he says. Whatever the acupuncture was doing, it wasn't working as a placebo.

It was the first hint, says Harris, that the central tenet of placebo-controlled trials – that placebo effects are always the same regardless of whether patients receive a real or fake treatment – might be wrong. 'It has been assumed by the pain community that the placebo effect should be embedded in the active treatment group,' he says. 'But it looks like actually placebos just do something completely different from the actual treatment … Both things are not necessarily operating together.'

Harris thinks that rather than representing a drop in endorphin levels, his results reveal an increase in the overall number of receptors. Other researchers have found that stimulating isolated neurons (nerve cells) directly causes extra opioid receptors to be expressed on the surface of those cells. Harris speculates that stimulating patients' nerves with

acupuncture needles might have a similar effect.

If he's right, it's tantalising evidence that while placebo acupuncture eases short-term symptoms by triggering pain-relieving endorphins, the real thing might actually help to reverse the underlying pathology of a disease. For example, fibromyalgia patients have fewer opioid receptors than healthy volunteers, leaving them less responsive to endorphins and overly sensitive to pain, but in Harris' study, acupuncture 'seemed to normalise the values back to healthy control levels,' he says. The larger that change, the more patients' pain fell.

Harris is seeking funding to follow up on his results, including testing whether fibromyalgia patients who receive true acupuncture do better long term.

More recently, research from Harvard Medical School has raised similar questions. A series of studies led by Vitaly Napadow, a neuroscientist at the Martinos Center for Biomedical Imaging at Massachusetts General Hospital and Harvard Medical School, also concluded that patients' initial pain ratings can hide important differences. He tested a therapy called electro-acupuncture, in which a mild electric current is passed through the needles.

Napadow focused on carpal tunnel syndrome, in which a squeezed nerve at the wrist causes numbness and pain. Unlike many chronic pain disorders, carpal tunnel syndrome is associated with physiological changes that can be measured objectively – nerve impulses at the wrist travel more slowly, for example.

In a randomised controlled trial published in March, 80 patients received either real electro-acupuncture or a fake version (in which retractable needles were placed at non-acupuncture points, with no electric current), in 16 sessions over eight weeks. Immediately after the treatment, all the patients reported similar reductions in their symptoms. Scientists would normally conclude from this result that the acupuncture didn't work. But as in Harris' trials, the underlying physiological effects were very different. The

true acupuncture groups showed measurable improvements in the speed of nerve transmission and in the somatosensory cortex that weren't seen in the placebo group. And only the true acupuncture groups still had reduced pain after three months. The larger the physiological changes measured by the team immediately after treatment, the better the patients felt three months later.

For MacPherson, the acupuncture advocate from the University of York, that's a compelling result. 'He's showing changes in the brain in response to acupuncture that are clearly linked to the person's improving clinical symptoms,' he says. MacPherson cautions that decisions regarding whether acupuncture should be prescribed to patients must always be based on clinical improvements in trials, not mechanistic studies, but he describes Harris and Napadow as 'pioneers', arguing that research like this is important for understanding how acupuncture might work, and suggesting how clinical trials could be better designed to pick up its effects.

These are single studies, however, and not everyone is convinced. 'I think there is nothing that can't be explained by bad statistical practice and cherry picking of evidence,' says Colquhoun. He describes Harris and Napadow's research as the sort of thing that merits the hashtag neurobabble (or even neurobollocks). 'Looking for explanations of a phenomenon before there's any proven phenomenon to investigate is a waste of time,' he insists.

But Harris is unfazed, arguing that regardless of the sceptics, wider opinion is moving towards an acceptance of acupuncture. 'Some people are not willing to change, despite the evidence,' he says. 'But gradually, we are seeing a shift.'

7 September 2017

⇨ The above information is reprinted with kind permission from *The Guardian*. Please visit www.theguardian.com for further information.

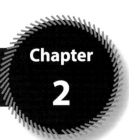

Why people use complementary or alternative therapies

here are a number of reasons why people use complementary or alternative therapies.

An overview of studies (a meta analysis) published in 2012 suggested that around half of people with cancer use some sort of complementary therapy at some time during their illness.

There is no evidence to suggest that any type of complementary therapy prevents or cures cancer.

For some therapies there is currently very little research evidence to show that they help with certain symptoms – for example, pain or hot flushes.

But there is research going on and we are starting to collect evidence for some types of therapy.

Using therapies to help you feel better

People often use complementary therapies to help them feel better and cope with having cancer and treatment. How you feel plays a part in how you cope.

Many complementary therapies concentrate on relaxation and reducing stress. They might help to calm your emotions, relieve anxiety, and increase your general sense of health and well-being.

Many doctors, cancer nurses and researchers are interested in the idea that positive emotions can improve your health.

Reducing symptoms or side effects

There is growing evidence that certain complementary therapies can help to

control some symptoms of cancer and treatment side effects.

For example, acupuncture can help to relieve sickness caused by some chemotherapy drugs. Or, it can help relieve a sore mouth after having treatment for head and neck cancer.

Acupuncture can also help to relieve pain after surgery to remove lymph nodes in the neck.

Feeling more in control

Sometimes it might feel as though your doctor makes many of the decisions about your treatment. It can feel like you don't have much control over what happens to you.

Many people say complementary therapy lets them take a more active role in their treatment and recovery, in partnership with their therapist.

Natural and healing therapies

Many patients like the idea that complementary therapies seem natural and non-toxic.

Some complementary therapies can help with specific symptoms or side effects. But we don't know much about how they might interact with conventional treatments like cancer drugs or radiotherapy.

And some types of complementary or alternative medicine might make conventional treatment work less well. And some might increase side effects.

Comfort from touch, talk and time

Some people might get a lot of comfort and satisfaction from the touch,

talk and time that a complementary therapist usually offers.

A good therapist can play a supportive role during cancer treatment and recovery. For example, a skilled and caring aromatherapist can take the time to make you feel cared for. This might help improve your quality of life.

Staying positive

Having a positive outlook is an important part of coping with cancer for most people. It is normal to want and hope for a cure, even if your doctor suggests that this might be difficult.

Some people use complementary therapies as a way to feel positive and hopeful for the future.

Boosting your immune system

There are claims that certain complementary therapies can boost their immune system and help fight cancer. There is evidence that feeling good and reducing stress boosts the immune system. But doctors don't know if this can help the body to control cancer.

There are clinical trials looking at how certain complementary therapies might affect the immune system.

Looking for a cure

Some people believe that using specific alternative therapies instead of conventional cancer treatment might help control or cure their cancer. There are also people who promote alternative therapies in this way.

Using alternative therapy can become more important to people with advanced cancer if their conventional treatment is no longer helping to control it. It is understandable that they hope that alternative therapies might work.

But, there is no scientific evidence to prove that any type of alternative therapy can help to control or cure cancer. Some alternative therapies might be unsafe and can cause harmful side effects.

20 March 2018

⇨ The above content is supplied by the world's largest charitable funder of cancer research, Cancer Research UK. Please visit www.cancerresearchuk.org for further information.

Homeopathy: what you need to know about the controversial alternative medicine

By Richard Jones

As a protest march against the use of homeopathic remedies to treat pets descended on Westminster earlier this week, Professor Edzard Ernst ignited a 13-year row with monarch-to-be Prince Charles over the latter's support of homeopathy.

Prince Charles has been a vocal supporter of homeopathy for decades, making impassioned speeches at the World Health Assembly and British Medical Association. However, Professor Ernst, who has previously labelled Prince Charles a 'snake oil salesman', said homeopathic treatments were 'immoral' and warned that royal backing was 'very worrying'.

Professor Ernst said: 'You can't have alternative medicine just because Prince Charles likes it, because that is not in the best interest of the patients.

'The quality of the research is not just bad, but dismal. It ignores harms. There is a whole shelf of rubbish being sold and that is simply unethical.'

So, what does this homeopathy business actually entail? And does it work?

The alternative medical practice of homeopathy is normally said to have been founded in 1796 by German physician Samuel Hahnemann (although some claim that Hippocrates started the ball rolling over 2,000 years ago). Hahnemann coined the mantra 'like cures like' – the belief that a substance that causes certain

---

> ### Four common homeopathic remedies
>
> **Allium cepa (onion):** As onions are known to make your eyes and nose runny, they are used in the treatment of hay fever and common colds.
>
> **Nux vomica (poison nut):** A toxic substance found in the seeds of the poison-nut tree, too much Nux vomica can cause liver failure. It is used in the treatment of mal impotence and hangovers.
>
> **Rhus tox (poison ivy):** This poisonous plant is known for growing everywhere – up walls and trees or across uncovered ground. This restless characteristic makes it a commonly proposed remedy among those suffering from restlessness and joint pain.
>
> **Chamomilla (camomile):** A commonly used homeopathic treatment in subduing restless children.

---

symptoms can also help to remove those symptoms.

Hahnemann struck upon this revelation while translating a book by Scottish chemist William Cullen. The book ascribed the usefulness of Peruvian bark in treating malaria due to its supposed astringent and bitter qualities, an explanation Hahnemann disputed seeing as there were many more substances more astringent and bitter than Peruvian bark that had no affect on treating malaria.

To test the hypothesis, Hahnemann consumed an inordinate amount of toxic Peruvian bark – a process in homeopathy called 'proving' – that gave him a high fever and chills similar to malaria. He decided that because the bark gave him – a healthy person – the same symptoms as malaria, it would therefore cancel out the symptoms were he to take it when he had the illness.

As munching on a load of Peruvian bark is likely to make anyone sick –

malaria or no malaria – Hahnemann had to figure out a way of prescribing low doses without causing everyone to break out into multiplying chills. Here we encounter the second principle of homeopathy: succussion. This is how medicines in homeopathy are made – by diluting substances in alcohol or distilled water and than shaking them violently, activating the 'vital energy' in the 'medicine', according to Hahnemann.

From this, Hahnemann decreed that the more diluted and weakened a substance was, the more potent it became.

Historically, the medical profession has had a hard time grappling with this logic. David Robert Grimes, a physicist at Oxford University, wrote in 2012 that Hahnemann's dilution decree was 'the antithesis of what is observed in nature, where the potency of any solution is proportional to the active ingredient in that substance.'

At such low amounts it begs the questions whether the treatment merely creates a placebo effect, an opinion that has been suggested by countless studies on the subject. In a 2010 report, the House of Commons Science and Technology Committee said there is no evidence that homeopathy is effective as a treatment for any health condition. The report called homeopathy's 'like cures like' principle 'theoretically weak', and said that this is the 'settled view of medical science'.

In the same year, hundreds of sceptics held protests outside Boots stores around the country against the pharmacy chain's decision to stock homeopathic products. The protestors swallowed whole bottles of homeopathic pills, overdosing on the recommended amounts. No hospitalisations were reported in the aftermath.

The British Medical Association calls homeopathy 'witchcraft', while the NHS says, 'there is no good-quality evidence that homeopathy is effective as a treatment for any health condition'.

Not all the evidence is negative. There have been trials showing the positive effects of homeopathic remedies in the treatment of hay fever, diarrhoea and ear infections among children. Members of the wider medical community have criticised the homeopathic industry for supposedly 'cherry-picking' facts in order to support their arguments.

And while homeopathic treatments are generally seen as harmless – as the mass overdose in 2010 suggested – the concern is that believers in the practice will eschew other scientifically grounded medicines. As such, the recommended course of action for anyone experiencing new symptoms remains a visit to the local GP.

18 January 2018

⇨ The above information is reprinted with kind permission from *The Telegraph*. Please visit www.telegraph.co.uk for further information.

Are complementary therapies safe during pregnancy?

In general, you should avoid taking any unnecessary medicines or treatments when you're pregnant. There are very few high-quality studies into the effectiveness of complementary or 'alternative' treatments, and anything you take into your body can affect your unborn baby.

What are complementary therapies?

Complementary medicines and treatments include a wide range of treatments that are not usually used by most doctors in the UK. These treatments are sometimes described as alternative medicine. However, 'complementary' is a better description, as they should be used alongside, but never replace, the treatment offered by your doctor.

Few complementary or alternative medicines are known to be safe during pregnancy. And some herbal remedies, such as blue cohosh, can actually be harmful for the baby.

But there is some evidence to support the use of:

⇨ massage and aromatherapy for treating anxiety

⇨ acupressure and ginger for morning sickness.

There are still times during pregnancy when they may not be safe. For example, your abdomen should not be massaged during the first three months of pregnancy.

Get medical advice

If you're considering using a complementary therapy, it's important to tell your GP or midwife about what treatment you're considering. If you then decide to use a complementary therapy, you should always consult a qualified practitioner.

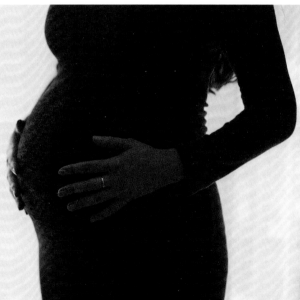

Complementary and alternative medicine can't replace conventional antenatal care. It's important to attend regular antenatal check-ups throughout your pregnancy.

23 May 2018

⇨ The above information is reproduced with kind permission from the NHS. Please visit www.nhs.uk for further information.

Acupuncture is effective for relieving period pain

The findings of a new study have shown that the intensity and duration of period pain can be reduced by up to 50 per cent by administering manual acupuncture.

By Maria Cohut

Period pain, or dysmenorrhea, is a condition affecting up to 95 per cent of menstruating women, according to a report published in the journal *Human Reproduction Update*.

Dysmenorrhea is classified into two types: primary, wherein no known health conditions can account for the painful cramps, and secondary, during which the pain occurs as a result of a diagnosed disorder, such as endometriosis or uterine fibroids.

A new study led by Australian researchers tests the effectiveness of acupuncture treatments in relieving period pain.

The study was conducted by Dr Mike Armour, of the National Institute of Complementary Medicine (NICM) at Western Sydney University in Australia, and his colleagues from the Department of Obstetrics and Gynaecology at the University of Auckland, also in Australia. Their findings were published in the journal *PLOS One*.

Frequent sessions most effective

74 adult women aged between 18 and 45 were involved in the study. They all had confirmed or suspected primary dysmenorrhea, and no diagnosis leading to the detection of secondary dysmenorrhea.

The women were randomly split into four groups: two high-frequency groups and two low-frequency groups. One-high frequency and one low-frequency group were assigned manual acupuncture treatments, with the remaining two undergoing electroacupuncture, wherein the needles are connected to a device that transmits electric impulses to the body.

The participants in the high-frequency groups received three acupuncture treatments one week prior to the start of their menstrual period. Meanwhile, the women in the low-frequency groups received three treatments every seven to ten days, between their menstrual periods.

All participants were administered 12 acupuncture treatments over three menstrual cycles. They also underwent a treatment in the first 48 hours of their menstrual period.

It was found that the women undergoing acupuncture more frequently experienced more significant improvements in period pain intensity and related symptoms, as well as in overall quality of life.

The researchers do acknowledge, however, that larger trials are needed if specialists are to develop detailed, accurate guidelines for the use of acupuncture in the treatment of this complaint.

Pragmatic trials of acupuncture have shown a reduction in pain intensity and an improvement in quality of life in women with period pain; however, evidence has been limited for how changing the 'dosage' of acupuncture might affect the outcome, says Dr Armour.

Manual or electroacupuncture?

All the participants involved in the study were asked to keep a diary providing details about the development of their menstrual period symptoms throughout the trial.

The researchers were surprised to find that more than half the women undergoing manual acupuncture experienced a decrease in period pain and related symptoms of up to 50 per cent.

This made manual acupuncture significantly more effective in treating

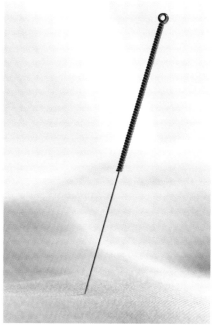

period pain than electroacupuncture, overall.

All the treatments administered over the course of the study conformed to a manualised protocol relying on data collected from a survey of specialised acupuncturists from Australia and New Zealand, alongside focus groups.

The treatment was grounded in traditional Chinese medicine practices as well as the zang fu system, which identifies the unique attributes of each organ and the ways in which they relate to each other.

Dr Armour and colleagues' findings are intriguing, and they may point to a new treatment for women seeking to minimise the impact of dysmenorrhea on their lives.

21 July 2017

⇨ The above information is reprinted with kind permission from Medical News Today. Please visit www.medicalnewstoday.com for further information.

Fibromyalgia sufferers see chronic pain symptoms reduced in new meditation therapy study

A team of academics has conducted the first study into the effectiveness of compassion meditation for treating fibromyalgia, a debilitating pain condition, which recently hit the headlines for causing Lady Gaga to cancel her world tour.

The study, which compared Attachment-based Compassion Therapy (ABCT) with relaxation techniques for treating fibromyalgia, was assessed by researchers from the University of Derby, the Awake to Wisdom Centre for Meditation and Mindfulness Research in Italy, and the Primary Care Prevention and Health Promotion Research Network, University of Zaragoza and Parc Sanitari Sant Joan de Déu in Spain.

As the chronic pain disorder affects approximately three per cent of adults in the UK and Europe with more women diagnosed than men, the team ran the study trial among 42 diagnosed women, split into two groups.

Compared to the relaxation control group, participants in the compassion therapy group demonstrated significant improvements across a range of psychological outcomes and reduced fibromyalgia symptoms by 36 per cent overall.

Dr William Van Gordon, Lecturer in Psychology at University of Derby Online Learning, said: 'The effectiveness of pharmacological treatments for fibromyalgia, such as anti-depressants, has long been questioned and can lead to unwanted side effects. The aim of this study was to investigate the use of compassion meditation as an alternative treatment for fibromyalgia.'

'Following the study, most participants in the ABCT group showed significant improvements and some no longer

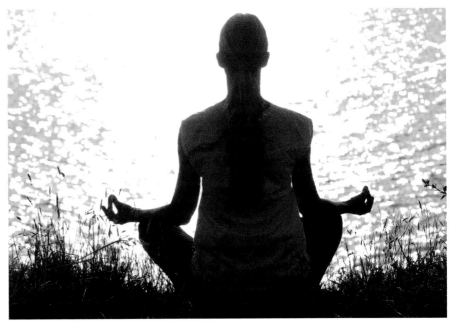

met the diagnostic criteria for fibromyalgia.

'As fibromyalgia is linked with sickness-related absence from work, incapacity to work, reduced work productivity and high usage of health-care resources, these results are not only meaningful for the sufferers but could help to address the problem of absence from work and the cost implications of this.'

The compassion therapy involved group sessions and daily homework assignments. Compassion meditation exercises were used to focus on cultivating a recognition and understanding of the universality of suffering, an emotional connection with others' suffering, and motivation to act to alleviate suffering.

Fibromyalgia symptoms were measured before and after the trial using the *Fibromyalgia Impact Questionnaire* (FIQ), an instrument developed to assess the current health status of women with fibromyalgia syndrome in clinical and research settings.

Before the start of trial, both the compassion therapy group and

control group had an FIQ average score of over 60. A score of 59 or more corresponds to a severe level of fibromyalgia symptoms. After the trial, the average score for the mediation group fell to 44, but the average score for the control group remained above 60.

While some symptoms were still likely to be present for participants in the ABCT group, they no were longer deemed to be severe. A reduction of at least 14 per cent is deemed to be clinically important, but in this study the reduction in symptoms was in the order of 3 per cent for fibromyalgia, 3 per cent for psychological flexibility, 4 per cent for anxiety, 5 per cent for depression, and 38 per cent for quality of life.

2018

⇨ The above information is reprinted with kind permission from the University of Derby. Please visit www.derby.ac.uk for further information.

It's better to curse when you feel pain, say scientists who swear by new research

The next time you bash your thumb with a hammer, yelling out a swear word could help you relieve pain, scientists say.

By Staff Reporter

It's always felt therapeutic to yell out a curse when you've accidentally bashed your thumb with a hammer or crashed into something. Now scientists have claimed a hell-raising, four-letter cry is the best form of pain relief.

Though older people may frown upon the use of coarse language, swearing can actually raise your tolerance to periods of agony.

A study in which – foolhardy – volunteers allowed themselves to undergo pain found that those who fell back on impolite language could withstand discomfort for twice as long as those who chose to grin and bear it.

The researchers from the universities of Keele and Central Lancashire assessed people from Britain, and Japan, where cursing in public is frowned upon much more than in the UK.

All of the participants were told to put their 'non-dominant' hand in icy water, the *Mail on Sunday* reported.

One-half were told to 'repeatedly' curse, either in Japanese or English, while the others use more polite language.

The British cursers were able to keep their hands in the water for 78.8 seconds compared to those who didn't at 45.7. The Japanese, meanwhile, had a far lower tolerance. Those who swore kept their hand in for 55.6 seconds, while those who didn't lasted for 25.4 seconds.

It is understood that swearing provokes an emotional response leading to what is described as a 'stress-induced analgesia', also known as the 'fight or flight' response, along with a surge of adrenaline.

Reporting in the imaginatively-titled *Scandinavian Journal of Pain*, the researchers said: 'Individuals from both Japanese and British cultures were more tolerant of the painful stimulus when swearing – this was not expected.

'Swearing could be encouraged as an intervention to help people cope with acute painful stimuli.'

In line with this foul-mouthed news we have put together a list of interesting swearing facts...

⇨ *The movie with the most swear words ever – Summer of Sam (1999)*

Spike Lee's take on the 'Son of Sam' murders in New York City during the summer of 1977 uses the word 'f**k' a total of 435 times throughout the film.

⇨ *We swear a lot*

According to analysis of spoken conversations, approximately 80–90 spoken words each day – 0.5% to 0.7% of all words – are swear words, with usage varying from between 0% to 3.4%. In comparison, first-person plural pronouns (we, us, our) make up 1% of spoken words.

⇨ *The first person to swear on British national television – Kenneth Tynan (1965)*

Critic and author Kenneth Tynan sparked outrage when he became the first person to say the F-word on British television.

27 August 2017

⇨ The above information is reprinted with kind permission from the *International Business Times*. Please visit www.ibtimes.co.uk for further information.

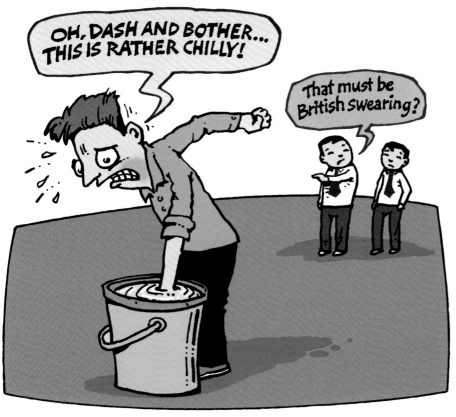

OH, DASH AND BOTHER... THIS IS RATHER CHILLY!

That must be British swearing?

How 'giggle doctors' help sick children

An article from **The Conversation.**

THE CONVERSATION

By Caspar Addyman, Lecturer in Developmental Psychology, Goldsmiths University of London

Hospitals are not fun for any of us. But imagine being trapped in a hospital bed as a young child, perhaps with a serious condition that requires multiple extended visits. Staff on children's wards do their best to entertain their patients but their first priority, of course, is always medical.

This is where 'giggle doctors' come in. These professional entertainers are trained and paid to go round hospitals to cheer up children with music and laughter. As a researcher interested in the benefits of laughter, I am fascinated by the work giggle doctors do and how it might make a difference to sick and disabled children. But as a scientist I am also challenged as to how we might measure these effects.

Every year there are around one million hospital admissions of children under 15, many of them serious and extended. With their tiny team of just 25 giggle doctors, Theodora Children's Charity is able to visit 33,000 of these children each year. Each visit has the potential to make a difference. As one parent told the charity, thanks to a giggle doctor, her daughter 'actually looks forward to coming to hospital for chemotherapy'.

In a typical visit a giggle doctor may see 25 children, spending about ten minutes with each one. In a year one giggle doctor will visit over 1,000 children. They are not medical professionals but the charity provides them with training in how to interact with poorly and disabled children and how to work best with doctors and nurses.

They currently visit 21 hospitals, three hospices and two specialist care centres throughout England and feedback shows that hospitals believe that they improve children's experience of hospital. But so far there has not been any systematic research to assess how they help children. The charity do keep good records of their team's work but they have not got systematic data. Part of the reason is that the benefits are intangible.

Giggle doctors are actors, entertainers, musicians and magicians. Laughter is important, but there is more to it than that. Every other interaction with an adult in a hospital is transactional. Giggle doctors do not using humour to distract from some unpleasant procedure; they are an escape and a respite. The emphasis is on connection and attention.

Clare Parry Jones, known to children as Dr Ding Dong, has been a giggle doctor for 18 years. Interviewed by the BBC she said: 'I have learned to celebrate the time I have with each child … It's a gift to be able to go in able to spend time with people and not care about anything else except for them.'

What's the science say?

I'm not a giggle doctor, but a child psychologist. I know children with serious medical conditions do not stop being children, and as a laughter researcher I know that the secret of any good performance is to know your audience and be able to connect with them. Which is why Dr Ding Dong's repertoire includes lots of jokes about poo.

But scientific research on the health benefits of laughter has been surprisingly thin on the ground. There is evidence of laughter's physiological benefits. Robin Dunbar and colleagues showed in 2011 that laughter can increase our pain threshold and recent research has show that this is because laughter stimulates the release of the endogenous opioids, the body's own painkillers. Other research with adults suggests laughter can improve vascular function and increase serotonin levels.

The closest fit in the research literature are two small pilot studies. Margaret Stuber, a child psychiatrist based at UCLA, has worked with US charity programme Rx Laughter™, which aims to promote comedy in a therapeutic setting. In 2007 they asked children to watch funny videos before, during

or after putting their hand in very cold water. The amount of laughter didn't change their pain tolerance, but children did keep their hand in the water longer while distracted by the video. Only 18 children were tested however and Stuber herself describes it as a pilot study.

Meanwhile, in 2011, a group at Holland Bloorview Kids Rehabilitation Hospital in Toronto, Canada, saw how 13 children with disabilities responded to two therapeutic clowns as compared to a control of watching television. The study measured physiological and emotional responses, but the results were a bit of a mess. Children's moods certainly improved but the physiological data showed no clear patterns and again the sample size was tiny.

None of this research directly addresses the effectiveness of the giggle doctors or gets at the holistic benefits their visits seem to bring. But the many thousands of visits they make offer a tremendous opportunity for research. It's not clear, however, how we might conduct a gold-standard randomised control trial on the work of the giggle doctors. Do we send in control performers who are trained not to be funny? Finding funding is also challenging for studies that are seemingly a frivolous luxury.

But should laughter be considered a frivolous luxury? Feedback from parents suggests the visits reduced stress and anxiety, and measuring the impact of such programmes will be important for their expansion. Although perhaps the real benefits are more intangible: found in those magic moments.

27 March 2018

⇨ The above information is reprinted with kind permission from *The Conversation*. Please visit www.theconversation.com for further information.

Drilling holes in the skull was never a migraine cure – here's why it was long thought to be

An article from The Conversation.

THE CONVERSATION

By Katherine Foxhall, Lecturer in History, University of Leicester

Trepanation – the technique of removing bone from the skull by scraping, sawing, drilling or chiselling – has long fascinated those interested in the darker side of medical history. One stock tale is that trepanning is one of the most ancient treatments for migraines. As I study the history of the migraine, it certainly has always caught my attention.

The word trepanation comes from the Greek trypanon, meaning a borer. The earliest known trepanned skulls date from around 10,000 BCE, and come from North Africa. There are trepanation accounts in the Hippocratic texts (5th century BCE), when it was used in cases of fracture, epilepsy or paralysis, and in the second century CE Galen wrote of his experiments with trepanation on animals in his clinical studies.

But the reasons for trepanning remain largely unknown. While the famous 17th-century physician William Harvey may have suggested that the procedure was used for migraines, recent authors have acknowledged that there is little evidence to suggest this. So where did this persistent idea come from?

Migraines and fairies

The real source of the myth seems to have come much later. In 1902, the *Journal of Mental Science* published a lecture by Sir Thomas Lauder Brunton, a London physician well known for his work on pharmacology and ideas about migraine pathology. The lecture mixed neurological theory and armchair anthropology, and ranged over subjects including premonitions, telepathy, hypnotism, hallucinations, and epileptic and migrainous aura. In one notable passage, Brunton proposed that visions of fairies and the sound of their jingling bells were 'nothing more' than the zigzags of migraine aura, and the aural results of nerve centre stimulation.

Brunton proposed that openings bored into ancient Stone Age skulls during life had been made to cure migraine. His suggestion followed considerable excitement during the 1870s when the French physician and anthropologist Paul Broca claimed that ancient skulls discovered in Peru and France had not only been opened surgically during life in order to release evil spirits, but that the patients had survived. To Brunton, it seemed obvious that the holes would have been made at the request of migraine sufferers in order to 'let the headache out'. He wrote:

'For when the pain of headache becomes almost unbearably severe, an instinctive desire sometimes arises either to strike the place violently in the hope of relieving the pain, or to wish that some operation could be done to remove the pain.'

The French surgeon Just Lucas-Championnière had claimed in 1878 that some South Sea islanders still performed a similar procedure but, essentially, Brunton's ideas about trepanning were as imaginative as his thoughts on fairies.

Nevertheless, the theory gained traction. In 1913, the world-famous American physician William Osler repeated that trepanation operations had been used 'for epilepsy, infantile convulsions, headache and various cerebral diseases believed to be caused by confined demons'. By 1931, T Wilson Parry (who was partial to the odd experiment of his own) reasoned in *The Lancet* that as the large numbers of trepanned skulls found throughout France could not all be accounted for by epilepsy, the procedure must also have been used to cast out 'other devils'. He proposed that this included disorders with 'exasperating' head symptoms such as migraine, giddiness, 'and distracting noises of the head'.

A 'burr hole'

If Victorian theories about ancient trepanation for migraine were largely speculative, there is evidence of cutting holes in skulls for migraine somewhat closer to home. In 1936, Alfred Goltman, a physician from Tennessee, observed something strange about a woman with migraine that he was treating for allergies.

In the left frontal region of her skull, the woman had a depression, an inch in diameter, with a marked concentration of blood vessels. Four years earlier, she had been admitted to the care of Dr Raphael Eustace Semmes, the first neurosurgeon in Memphis, who had trained under Harvey Cushing, the American 'father' of modern neurosurgery. Semmes had drilled a small circular opening known as a 'burr hole' during one of the woman's severe headaches, while she was under local anaesthetic. As he opened the thick membrane surrounding the brain, 'a quantity of fluid escaped under increased pressure'. There was no evidence of a tumour.

This now seems a troubling era in experimental interventionist neurosurgery. Between the 1890s and the 1920s, some surgeons believed that brain surgery could 'cure' inherited criminal tendencies. Children referred by juvenile courts were operated on in an attempt to release 'pressure on the brain', a procedure with a mortality rate of up to 42%. By the 1930s, frontal lobotomy was emerging as a treatment for mental illness.

Semmes' patient survived the surgery, but her migraine headaches did not stop. Goltman noticed that during her headaches the depression left by the surgery began to fill up. As the migraine attack ended, the swelling would recede. Goltman's observations helped influence the widespread acceptance of a theory that would dominate understanding of migraine until the 1970s: that the origin of migraine headache must be vascular,

characterised by dilation of the blood vessels during the attack.

While we now see migraine as neurological, much still remains to be discovered about its causes and mechanisms in the brain. In some ways, trepanning does seem a logical response to the intense pain of migraine. As Andrew Levy notes in his memoir: 'The migraining head wants to be cut open; it longs to be cut open.' This does not, of course, mean that it should be.

6 March 2018

⇨ The above information is reprinted with kind permission from *The Conversation*. Please visit www.theconversation.com for further information.

Review highlights the danger of mixing herbal remedies with prescription drugs

'**M**illions of people could be risking their health by taking herbal remedies and prescription drugs at the same time, scientists warn,' is the front-page headline in the *Daily Mail*.

Researchers from South Africa reviewed instances of potential interactions between conventional drugs and herbal remedies, and found a wide range of dangers.

Looking at 49 reports of possible adverse reactions, they determined that 59% were probably caused by interactions between prescription drugs and herbal remedies. They also found two studies showing an additional 15 cases of drug-herb reactions.

Herbal remedies can affect the way drugs act on the body, either blocking their action or increasing their potency. Problems reported in the review included liver and kidney damage, bleeding, nausea, vomiting and diarrhoea, mental health problems, seizures and muscle pain.

Many combinations of drugs and herbal remedies caused interactions, but the most commonly mentioned drugs were warfarin and statins.

The review underlines the importance of telling your doctor that you're taking herbal remedies if you're prescribed

a drug – just because a substance is described as a herb, that doesn't mean it's harmless or safe for everyone to use.

Some people are embarrassed to admit they're taking herbal remedies, but it's vital you tell your doctor or pharmacist.

Where did the story come from?

The study was carried out by researchers from the South African Medical Research Council and Stellenbosch University in South Africa. It was published in the peer-reviewed *British Journal of Clinical Pharmacology* on an open-access basis so is free to read online. No funding information was reported.

The *Daily Mail*, *The Guardian* and *The Sun* all gave a good overview of the study and its findings.

What kind of research was this?

This was a systematic review of case reports and observational studies containing descriptions of herb-drug interactions.

Systematic reviews are a good way to get an overview of the state of research on a topic. However, their overall quality depends on the strength of the studies included, and case reports are not a particularly reliable source of evidence.

What did the research involve?

Researchers looked for published evidence about herb-drug interactions – whether from clinical studies, observational studies or single-case reports – from January 2001 to August 2017

Using two scoring systems, they assessed how likely it was that the herb-drug interaction caused the reported problem, looked at potential mechanisms through which it might have occurred, and evaluated how many case reports showed a 'very probable', 'probable', 'possible' or 'doubtful' drug interaction. They also presented results from two additional observational studies that contained reports of drug-herb interactions.

The scoring systems used were Horn's Drug Interaction Probability Scale and the Roussel Uclaf Causality Assessment Method for liver damage.

What were the basic results?

The researchers found:

⇨ 49 case reports of drug-herb interactions, of which they said four were 'highly probable', 25 'probable', 18 'possible' and two 'doubtful'

⇨ Two observational studies of hospital inpatients, one from Israel and one from Korea – the Israeli

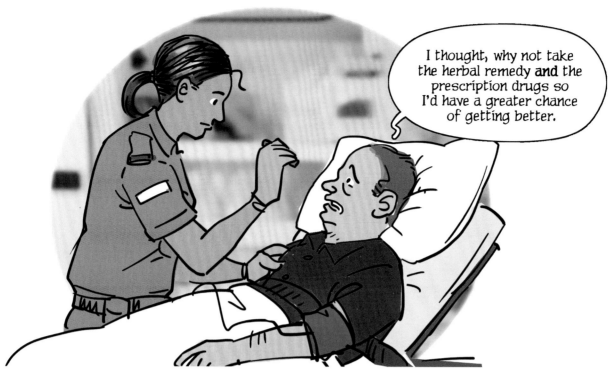

I thought, why not take the herbal remedy **and** the prescription drugs so I'd have a greater chance of getting better.

study reported nine drug-herb interactions among 947 patients, and the Korean study reported six drug-herb interactions among 313 patients.

Drugs affected included the blood-thinning drug warfarin, cholesterol-lowering statins, anti-cancer drugs, antidepressants, immunosuppressant drugs for organ transplants and antiretroviral drugs for people with HIV.

Herbal remedies included *Ginkgo Biloba*, St John's wort, ginseng, sage, flaxseed, cranberry, goji juice, green tea, chamomile and turmeric.

The most common illness among patients who experienced a drug-herb interaction was cardiovascular disease. In these patients, interactions affecting warfarin or statins were most common. Herbs that interacted with these drugs included sage, flaxseed, St John's wort, cranberry, goji juice, green tea and chamomile.

Other conditions affected included cancer, kidney transplants, depression, schizophrenia, anxiety disorders and seizures. One man died after a herbal remedy prevented his anti-seizure medication from working properly, resulting in him drowning.

Many people in the case reports were taking a combination of herbs or herbal preparations and a combination of prescription drugs, making it difficult to know which herb might have been interacting with which drug.

How did the researchers interpret the results?

The researchers said their review showed that 'few cases of potential HDI [herb-drug interactions] have been documented in the literature despite the detrimental consequences of such interactions'.

They called for additional research to clarify how commonly used herbs can affect medicines, in order to 'inform drug regulatory agencies and pharmaceutical companies about the need to update information in package inserts of medicines'.

Conclusion

Many people believe herbal remedies are safe, so they think they don't need to inform their doctor that they're taking them. However, all medicines, herbal or conventional, can have side effects.

Herbal medicines are also known to affect how conventional drugs work. For example, St John's wort can be dangerous if taken with antidepressants and can stop the contraceptive pill from working.

This study shows that even commonly used herbs and spices, such as green tea and turmeric, can cause problems when combined with certain medicines. That's why, if you're taking conventional medicines, it's crucial to tell your doctor if you're taking or planning to take herbal medicines.

Your doctor can tell you whether the herb in question might interact with a drug or make a medical condition worse. Check the leaflets that come with your conventional medicines to see if they warn against taking herbal medicines alongside them. You can also ask a pharmacist for advice.

Find out more about herbal medicines. You can report any side effect or adverse reaction to a herbal medicine using the Yellow Card Scheme run by the Medicines and Healthcare products Regulatory Agency. This can help identify new side effects or risks associated with medicines, including herbal remedies.

26 January 2018

⇨ The above information is reproduced with kind permission from the NHS. Please visit www.nhs.uk for further information.

Natural doesn't mean safe – herbal medicines found to contain steroids

People who may have purchased Yiganerjing Cream are urged to discontinue use immediately as it contains an undisclosed steroid and two antifungal ingredients.

The Medicines and Healthcare products Regulatory Agency (MHRA) is warning people who may have purchased a 'natural' Chinese herbal medicine, Yiganerjing Cream, as a treatment for skin conditions to stop using it immediately as it has been found to contain an undisclosed steroid and two antifungal ingredients.

MHRA officials have been acting to stop the sale of this cream and have had it withdrawn from many websites and on-line market places but people may have purchased it in the past and still be using it.

Yiganerjing Cream is not a licensed medicine and has been marketed in the UK as a 'natural' Chinese herbal medicine for the treatment of a range of skin conditions, most commonly eczema, psoriasis and rosacea.

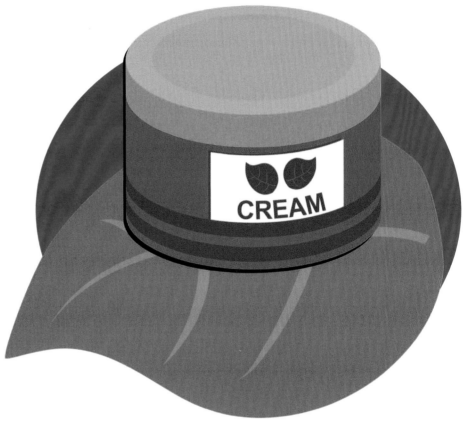

Our analysis found the presence of the steroid clobetasol propionate. This steroid is the active ingredient in prescription only medicines used for the treatment of a range skin conditions such as psoriasis and eczema. Creams containing steroids should be used sparingly and as directed by the prescriber. It is contraindicated in children under one year of age.

We are also aware of the use, via a herbal clinic, of a product called Penny Orange Cream which has also been found to contain clobetasol propionate. While this product is no longer available, and we are not aware of its widespread use, it did contain an undisclosed steroid and should not be used.

If you are unsure about the safety of a medicine claiming to be 'natural' or 'herbal' you should check for a Marketing Authorisation (MA) or Product Licence (PL) number or Traditional Herbal Registration (THR) number/the THR logo. This means the product has been assessed by MHRA for safety and has been manufactured correctly.

Dr Chris Jones, Manager of the Medicines Borderline Section at MHRA said:

'The sale of potent steroid creams directly to the public is illegal for good reason. If used without medical supervision these medicines can be dangerous.

'Steroids must be prescribed by healthcare professionals who follow strict criteria when prescribing them and monitoring patients using them.

They can suppress the skin's response to infection, can cause long-term thinning of the skin, and if applied long term over a wide area, particularly in babies and children, can cause other medical problems.

'Our advice to anyone who is using Yiganerjing Cream, particularly on young children and babies, is to discontinue use immediately. If you have any questions, please contact your healthcare professional.'

28 February 2018

⇨ The above information is reprinted with kind permission from Medicines and Healthcare products Regulatory Agency. Please visit www.gov.uk for further information.

NHS set to ban homeopathy for patients because it is 'not evidence based and any benefits are down to placebo'

Health service currently spends more than £90,000 a year on the natural treatment.

By Kate Forster, Health Correspondent

Doctors should stop prescribing homeopathic medicine to NHS patients, the health service has said. The change has been proposed because 'at best, homeopathy is a placebo and a misuse of scarce NHS funds which could better be devoted to treatments that work', said Simon Stevens, NHS England's chief executive.

The NHS currently spends £92,412 a year on the natural 'treatment', which uses highly diluted doses of natural substances that some claim help the body heal itself.

Recommendations set out in a consultation document categorise homeopathy as a treatment with a 'lack of robust evidence of clinical effectiveness' and say GPs should not give it to new patients in a drive to cut prescription costs.

Other treatments that could soon be banned by the NHS include herbal treatments, lidocaine plasters, omega-3 fatty acids and unlicensed use of the painkiller co-proxamol, which was withdrawn from the market in 2007 due to safety concerns. In March it was revealed that the cost-cutting plans could stop NHS doctors from providing travel vaccinations and prescriptions for hayfever tablets and gluten-free food for coeliacs.

'The NHS is probably the world's most efficient health service, but like every country there is still waste and inefficiency that we're determined to root out,' said Mr Stevens. 'The public rightly expects that the NHS will use every pound wisely, and today we're taking practical action to free up funding to better spend on modern drugs and treatments.'

The plans are at the centre of a formal public consultation aiming to save the health service at least £250 million a year.

Professor Helen Stokes-Lampard, chair of the Royal College of GPs, said it was appropriate to take 'safe, sensible measures' to reduce prescription costs, which are 'a significant expense for the health service'.

But she warned that forcing everyone to buy common medical items previously available on prescription risks 'alienating the most vulnerable in society'.

'We know that a number of treatments are of little or no value, and are at best a placebo,' she said. 'We also know many other medications are available very cheaply over the counter and are much more readily obtainable than when they first became available on prescription, and both GPs and the public should be mindful of this.

'If patients are in a position that they can afford to buy over-the-counter medicines and products, then we would encourage them to do so rather than request a prescription – but imposing blanket policies on GPs, that don't take into account demographic differences across the country, or that don't allow for flexibility for a patient's individual circumstances, risks alienating the most vulnerable in society.'

21 July 2017

⇨ The above information is reprinted with kind permission from *The Independent*. Please visit www.independent.co.uk for further information.

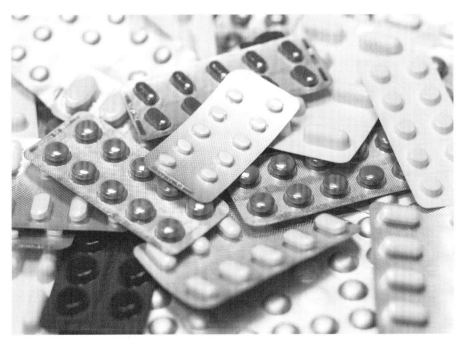

Why you can't trust homeopathy

It doesn't work

When tested under rigorous conditions – when neither the patient nor the doctor knows whether they're using homeopathy or not until all of the tests are done – homeopathy has shown to work no better than a sugar pill. That doesn't mean people do not feel better after taking homeopathy; only that those feelings aren't related to the homeopathy. This is known as the placebo effect and is often misunderstood. Conventional medicine also has a placebo effect, on top of its other benefits.

The choice between medicine and homeopathy comes down to a simple question: would you have a placebo, or a placebo plus a treatment that has been proven to work?

It couldn't work

The theoretical principles that underpin homeopathy lack any scientific credibility and the so-called 'laws of homeopathy' do not tally with anything we know about the world around us. Only a basic understanding of chemistry is needed to demonstrate that homeopathic tinctures can only be plain water.

It's a waste of your money

The homeopathy industry is worth around £40 million in the UK, and around €400 million in both France and Germany. While this may seem small compared to the pharmaceutical industry, pharmaceutical medicines are required to show clinical effectiveness before they are licensed for sale. Homeopathy bears no such requirements and £40 million is a lot of money to spend on something that you haven't proved works.

Homeopathic pills are being sold at a cost of around £5.95 for less than 20g of sugar pills. Without any active ingredient, that ultimately amounts to a lot of money for not a lot of sugar.

It's a waste of everyone's money

In the UK, the NHS spends an estimated £4 million every year on homeopathy. The British government also supports four homeopathic hospitals using taxpayers money, in Bristol, Glasgow, Liverpool and London. The evidence is very clear: homeopathy does not work and therefore has no place within the National Health Service. Despite the recent heavy cuts in public expenditure, the British Government still refuses to cut funding for homeopathy, even when advised to do so by top scientists.

It's a waste of your time

When homeopathy is accepted as a viable alternative to medicine, patients waste time taking useless pills and potions instead of seeking expert medical attention. For mild ailments, like a cough or a cold, the risks are minimal; but for patients with more severe conditions, time can be a significant factor in their recovery. Many homeopaths even directly encourage patients to wait before seeking medical attention, even when their condition deteriorates, claiming that worsening symptoms are a sign their potions are working.

Moreover, patients with terminal conditions are left with an unrealistic view of their condition and may be distracted from making the most of the time they have left. This ultimately leads to more heartache and suffering when the bogus treatment proves futile.

It's a waste of everyone's time

Thousands of studies have been conducted into the effectiveness of homeopathy and its various 'laws'. So far, none reliably shown homeopathy to be effective and most are conclusively negative. Any conventional treatment with a similar track record would have been dropped a long time ago. In fact, many treatments have been dropped, even with a stronger evidence base than exists for homeopathy. If we weren't wasting time proving, yet again, that homeopathy doesn't work, we could be looking for treatments that do.

There are alternatives to this alternative

The thing about homeopathy is, we don't need it. Medicine works. Diseases like measles, whooping cough and polio are effectively prevented by vaccination. Modern anti-retroviral drugs help HIV sufferers manage their condition so effectively that AIDS is no longer the death sentence it once was.

Homeopaths offer bogus 'cures' for AIDS, which leads to vulnerable people, sick to death, paying for the privilege.

It's not what it says on the label

Buy a vial of 30C homeopathic sulphur at your local pharmacy and one thing you can be sure you won't find in the bottle is any sulphur. You have significantly more chance of winning a triple rollover on the lottery than you have of finding even a single atom of sulphur in that tube; but the label still reads 'Sulphur'.

It detracts from medicine

Giving legitimacy to unproven and ineffective treatments does not come without a cost. The cost of allowing the promotion of homeopathy as an 'alternative' to medicine comes when patients are unable to distinguish between a self-limiting condition which will cure itself given time, and a more serious illness which will become life-threatening if incorrectly treated. Stories of people abandoning medicine in favour of quack cures, with disastrous results, are not hard to find. By allowing the promotion of a therapy proven to be ineffective and implausible, we encourage people to turn their back on the treatments that can help them.

It has abused its placebo privileges

From time to time, it's understandable that a simple-to-administer placebo treatment might carry some benefit for doctors, where no medical intervention has a particular, proven effectiveness. In these scenarios, it could be argued that homeopathy might have had a role to play, providing a harm-free, effect-free placebo to help manage the otherwise unmanageable. However, homeopaths abuse this minor level of legitimacy to make claims about conditions the placebo effect could not possible treat. Cancer, HIV, malaria, yellow fever, autism, tuberculosis. They discourage people from seeking medical help when they most need it. It's time to stop lending support to quackery; time to give people the facts about this 200-year-old snake oil, before they choose to use it instead of the ever-improving and reliable interventions of modern medicine.

⇨ The above information is reprinted with kind permission from 10:23. Please visit www.1023.org.uk for further information.

© 2018 The 10:23 Campaign

Top seven safe, effective natural antibiotics

Certain natural substances have antibacterial properties, but which are safe to use, and when should a person use them?

By Danielle Dresden

Reviewed by Debra Rose Wilson, PhD, MSN, RN, IBCLC, AHN-BC, CHT

Prescription antibiotics, such as penicillin, have helped people to recover from otherwise fatal diseases and conditions since the 1940s.

However, people are also turning to natural antibiotics for treatment.

According to the NHS, one in ten people experiences side effects that harm the digestive system after taking antibiotics. Around one in 15 people are allergic to this type of medication.

In this article, we look at the evidence behind seven of the best natural antibiotics. We also discuss which to avoid, and when to see a doctor.

Seven best natural antibiotics

The scientific jury is still out concerning natural antibiotics. While people have used remedies like these for hundreds of years, most treatments have not been thoroughly tested.

However, some show promising results under medical review, and further studies are underway.

With an ongoing increase in drug-resistant bacteria, scientists are looking to nature when developing new medications.

Here, we examine the science behind seven natural antibiotics.

1. Garlic

Cultures across the world have long recognised garlic for its preventive and curative powers.

Research has found that garlic can be an effective treatment against many forms of bacteria, including *Salmonella* and *Escherichia coli* (*E. coli*). Garlic has even been considered for use against multi-drug resistant tuberculosis.

2. Honey

Since the time of Aristotle, honey has been used as an ointment that helps wounds to heal and prevents or draws out infection.

Healthcare professionals today have found it helpful in treating chronic wounds, burns, ulcers, bedsores and skin grafts. For example, results of a study from 2016 demonstrate that honey dressings can help to heal wounds.

The antibacterial effects of honey are usually attributed to its hydrogen peroxide content. However, manuka honey fights off bacteria, though it has a lower hydrogen peroxide content.

A 2011 study reported that the best-known type of honey inhibits approximately 60 kinds of bacteria. It also suggests that honey successfully treats wounds infected with methicillin-resistant *Staphylococcus aureus* (MRSA).

Antibacterial properties aside, honey may help wounds to heal by providing a protective coating that fosters a moist environment.

3. Ginger

The scientific community also recognizes ginger as a natural antibiotic. Several studies, including one published in 2017, have demonstrated ginger's ability to fight many strains of bacteria.

Researchers are also exploring ginger's power to combat seasickness and nausea and to lower blood sugar levels.

4. Echinacea

Native American and other traditional healers have used *Echinacea* for hundreds of years to treat infections and wounds. Researchers are beginning to understand why.

A study published in the *Journal of Biomedicine and Biotechnology* reports that extract of *Echinacea purpurea* can kill many different kinds of bacteria, including *Streptococcus pyogenes* (*S. pyogenes*).

S. pyogenes is responsible for strep throat, toxic shock syndrome, and the 'flesh-eating disease' known as necrotizing fasciitis.

Echinacea may also fight inflammation associated with bacterial infection.

5. Goldenseal

Goldenseal is usually consumed in tea or capsules to treat respiratory and digestive problems. However, it may also combat bacterial diarrhoea and urinary tract infections.

In addition, results of a recent study support the use of goldenseal to treat skin infections. In a lab, goldenseal extracts were used to prevent MRSA from damaging tissue.

A person taking prescription medications should check with a doctor before taking goldenseal, as this supplement can cause interference.

Goldenseal also contains berberine, an important component of natural antibiotics. This alkaloid is not safe for infants, or women who are pregnant or breastfeeding.

6. Clove

Clove has traditionally been used in dental procedures. Research is now finding that clove water extract may be effective against many different kinds of bacteria, including *E. coli*.

7. Oregano

Some believe that oregano boosts the immune system and acts as an antioxidant. It may have anti-inflammatory properties.

While researchers have yet to verify these claims, some studies show that oregano is among the more effective natural antibiotics, particularly when it is made into an oil.

Risks of natural antibiotics

Just because something is labeled natural, it is not necessarily safe.

The amounts and concentrations of active ingredients vary among brands of supplements. Read labels carefully. A person should also inform their healthcare provider if they plan to take these supplements.

While cooked garlic is usually safe to consume, research suggests that taking concentrated garlic may increase the risk of bleeding. This can be dangerous for people facing surgery or taking blood thinners.

Garlic concentrates may also reduce the usefulness of HIV medications.

Certain products should be avoided, including colloidal silver. This substance consists of microscopic pieces of silver suspended in water.

Colloidal silver has been recommended as a treatment for a variety of diseases, including the bubonic plague and HIV. However, according to the National Center for Complementary and Integrative Health, it can be dangerous, and no credible studies back up these uses.

Taking colloidal silver supplements may interfere with the effectiveness of antibiotics and medication used to treat an underactive thyroid gland.

Silver can also build up in the body and turn the skin bluish-grey. This condition is called argyria and is permanent in most people.

When to use prescribed antibiotics

Due to the current increase in drug-resistant diseases, most doctors do not prescribe antibiotics unless they are effective and necessary.

Antibiotics are most often prescribed to:

⇨ prevent the spread of infectious diseases

⇨ prevent a condition from becoming more serious or fatal

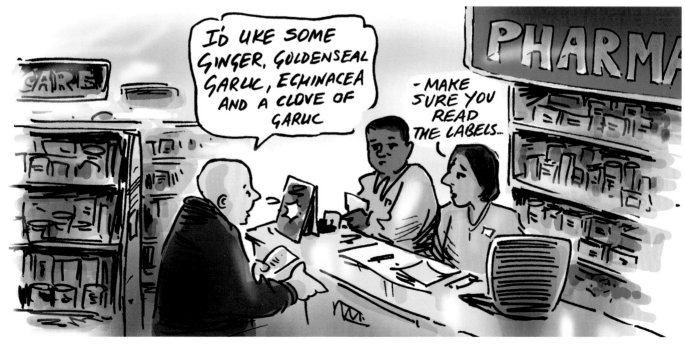

- speed recovery from illness or injury
- prevent development of complications.

If a person is prescribed antibiotics, they should take the entire dosage as directed. This is especially encouraged in people with a higher risk of bacterial infection, or who face greater risks if they become ill, such as people who are:

- scheduled for surgery
- receiving chemotherapy
- HIV-positive
- taking insulin for diabetes
- living with heart failure
- recovering from serious wounds

- over 75 years old
- under three days old

When an individual is allergic to prescription antibiotics or suffers side effects, they may want to discuss other options with a doctor.

Outlook

According to the Centers for Disease Control and Prevention (CDC), each year more than two million Americans become unwell from drug-resistant bacteria, resulting in 23,000 annual deaths.

These bacteria constitute a growing threat, and the key to developing new and effective medications may lie in treatments of the past – natural antibiotics.

While natural antibiotics may present opportunities, they also carry risks. Still, research into these treatments is growing, and an increasing number of substances are being tested. Natural antibiotics traditionally used for centuries may contribute to the lifesaving drugs of tomorrow.

3 March 2018

- The above information is reprinted with kind permission from Medical News Today. Please visit www.medicalnewstoday.com for further information.

Olive leaf benefits

Latin name

Olea europaea L. folium

Also known as

Olive leaf

Origin

Mediterranean Basin from Portugal to the Levant, the Arabian Peninsula, and southern Asia as far east as China

Parts used

Leaves

Traditional use and health Benefits

The olive leaf was so important to the Ancient Egyptians that they regarded it as a symbol of heavenly power. Not only did they extract the oil to mummify their kings, it was used as a powerful defender against a wide variety of maladies too.

This tree was so important it was referred to as the 'Tree of Life' in the Bible, held in such high esteem that Moses is said to have excluded olive tree growers from military service.

Fast forward to the 1880s when it was utilised to counteract malaria, and then in the early 1900s scientists isolated a bitter compound, 'oleuropein', that was thought to give the olive tree its disease resistance. And so through the later 1900s oleuropein was found to lower blood pressure in animals, increase blood flow in the coronary arteries, relieve arrhythmia and prevent internal muscle spasms.

Olive leaf benefits

Heart health

The first way olive leaf can benefit the heart is by its ability to foster significant drops in elevated blood pressure – extracts have been shown to both prevent and treat high blood pressure. One particularly fascinating study was conducted among identical twins with borderline hypertension (blood pressure in the range of 120–139 mmHg over 80–89 mmHg). Studies of identical twins virtually eliminate genetic variations which may impact study results. After eight weeks, placebo recipients showed no change in blood pressure from baseline, but patients supplemented with 1,000

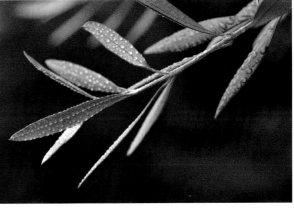

mg/day of olive leaf extract dropped their pressures by a mean of 11 mmHg systolic and four mmHg diastolic. The supplemented patients also experienced significant reductions in LDL cholesterol.

Secondly, olive leaf supports arterial health – the endothelial cells that line the arterial walls play a key role in maintaining blood flow and pressure, with endothelial dysfunction being one of the earliest stages of hardening of the arteries (atherosclerosis). Olive Leaf can fight endothelial dysfunction on many levels; it increases the production of nitric oxide – a signalling molecule that helps to relax blood vessels. This powerful leaf also has multi-targeted anti-inflammatory effects which may help to prevent the oxidisation of LDL cholesterol, which can damage arteries and, again, lead to atherosclerosis.

Finally, polyphenol compounds found in olive leaves have been shown to help directly prevent the formation of arterial plaques (and thereby reduce the risk of heart attack and stroke) in two ways. First, they reduce the production and activity of a series of 'adhesion molecules.' These substances cause white blood cells and platelets to stick to arterial walls, resulting in early plaque formation. Second, they reduce platelet aggregation (clumping) by multiple mechanisms, which in turn reduces the risk that tiny clots will form at sites of plaque to produce a stroke or heart attack.

Diabetes

There is evidence to suggest the olive leaf could provide a natural alternative for diabetes. Researchers from the University of Auckland have discovered extract of this leaf has the ability to decrease insulin resistance and increase the production of insulin by the pancreas.

In a randomised, double-blinded and placebo-controlled clinical study, the researchers found that the olive leaf extract lowered insulin resistance by an average of 15% and increased the productivity of the pancreas' beta cells – which produce insulin – by 28%.

This effect is due to the olive leaf's hypoglycaemic properties (lowers blood sugar in the body), and its ability to control blood glucose levels. The polyphenols in this leaf play a vital role in delaying the production of sugar, which is the precursor to inflammatory diseases such as diabetes.

Immune sytem

Olive leaves have been traditionally used for centuries to support the immune system, maintain overall good health and to relieve symptoms of coughs, colds and flu. It has five times (400%) more antioxidant power than the equivalent amount of vitamin C.

The olive leaf also has anti-viral properties with research showing that extracts can effectively fight against a number of disease-causing microbes. These powerful compounds destroy invading organisms and don't allow viruses to replicate and cause infection.

Anti-fungal

The aforementioned anti-microbial effect was tested in a 2003 study by D. Markin et al. The researchers found that olive leaf extracts killed almost all bacteria tested. This included dermatophytes which cause infections in the skin, hair and nails; *Candida albicans* – an agent of oral and genital infection, and *Escherichia coli* cells (*E. coli*) – bacteria found in the lower intestine.

This makes olive leaf a wonderful herb to eliminate *Candida* overgrowth, and an excellent anti-fungal for the treatment of athletes foot and toenail fungus.

Bone health

Inspired by epidemiological evidence showing that people who ate a traditional Mediterranean diet were less likely to suffer from osteoporosis, Dr Veronique Coxam has led research and development of the powerfully active compounds in olive leaf – oleuropein and hydroxytyrosol. Her early work found that both of these compounds had an impact on inflammation in bones – findings since confirmed by animal studies.

Research performed by scientists at the University of Cordoba, Spain, studied the effects of a range of oleuropein concentrations on the formation of osteoblasts (a cell that secretes the substance of bone), in stem cells from human bone marrow. The researchers concluded, 'Our data suggests that oleuropein, highly abundant in olive tree products included in the traditional Mediterranean diet, could prevent age-related bone loss and osteoporosis.'

Typical use

Use 30g of olive leaf per litre of water then boil until the water reduces to half the amount. Drink up to two cups

per day – one in the morning and one in the evening. Can be drunk hot or iced with a slice of lemon.

Folklore and history

Whilst anecdotal and biblical accounts of the olive leaf go back thousands of years, the first formal medical mention of the olive leaf occurred about 150 years ago – an account describing its ability to cure severe cases of fever and malaria. In 1854, *The Pharmaceutical Journal* contained a report by David Hanbury that included this simple healing recipe:

'Boil a handful of leaves in a quart of water down to half its original volume. Then administer the liquid in the amount of a wine glass every three to four hours until the fever is cured.'

The author said he discovered the tincture in 1943 and had used it successfully. His method became well known in England for treating the sick who were returning from the tropical colonies. He believed that a bitter substance in the leaves was the key healing ingredient – a fact now confirmed by modern science.

Constituents

Secoiridoids (oleuropein and its derivatives), hydroxytyrosol, polyphenols (verbascoside, apigenin-7-glucoside and luteolin-7-glucoside), triterpenes including oleanolic acid and flavonoids (rutin and diosmin).

Precautions

If you take any blood pressure medications or have low blood pressure, check with your health care professional before using olive leaf.

Not recommended if you are pregnant or breastfeeding.

⇨ The above information is reprinted with kind permission from Indigo Herbs. Please visit www.indigo-herbs.co.uk for further information.

© 2018 Indigo Herbs Ltd

More than 120 homeopaths trying to 'cure' autism in UK

Exclusive: the 'cure' involves detoxing children of vaccines and antibiotics held responsible for the condition.

By Sarah Boseley, Health Editor

More than 120 homeopaths in the UK are offering a 'cure' for autism that involves supposedly detoxing children of the vaccines and antibiotics held responsible for the condition, *The Guardian* has learned.

The homeopaths are accredited practitioners of CEASE 'therapy', which stands for Complete Elimination of Autistic Spectrum Expression. CEASE was invented by a Dutch doctor called Tinus Smits, who died of cancer in 2010.

His book and website, which lists therapists around the world, describe a method of ridding children of toxins – predominantly vaccines and medication – that are said to cause autism. It involves homeopathic remedies and high doses of vitamin C in excess of those recommended by national guidelines.

Diarrhoea, which could be a result of excessive vitamin C, and fever in children should not necessarily be cause for concern, say CEASE therapists, because it is the child's body purging itself of toxins.

'It's absolutely appalling,' said Carol Povey, director of the centre for autism at the National Autistic Society (NAS), which helps develop best practice. 'As healthcare practitioners, homeopaths should still be working on evidence-based practice and looking at national guidelines.'

The NAS is concerned by the suggestion that autism, a developmental disorder, could be cured. It is also disturbed by the claim that autism is linked to vaccines, as proposed by Andrew Wakefield – a theory that has been comprehensively discredited. Wakefield, a former gastroenterologist, was struck off the medical register over his claims.

Homeopathic cures, like other bogus therapies on the Internet, 'hoodwink new parents when they are vulnerable' and can cause harm, said Povey.

A minority of CEASE therapists in the UK are members of the Society of Homeopaths. Its regulatory body, the Professional Standards Authority (PSA), has said the Society of Homeopaths must state by the middle of next month what action it will take to ensure children are safe as a condition of its re-accreditation.

The PSA told the Society of Homeopaths that 'CEASE therapy contravenes medical advice by apparently advising against vaccination of children, avoiding antibiotics in the case of infection and advocates high doses of vitamins not recommended for children. We are also concerned that the full name of CEASE (Complete Elimination of Autistic Spectrum Expression) strongly implies the ability to cure autism through this therapy,' it said in a statement.

While the society had responded that its members 'should not be practising the aspects of CEASE that defy medical advice', this was not clear on its website, said the PSA.

Mark Taylor, chief executive of the Society of Homeopaths, said it was looking into how many of its members practised CEASE therapy and whether they complied with advice on respecting medical evidence. 'We are looking at the advice we will offer over the next few weeks so there is nothing more to say at the moment,' he told *The Guardian*.

Many other homeopaths who are also CEASE therapists are not members of the society. The PSA urges the public to choose only those on its accredited register.

Jennifer Hautman, a homeopath who is not a Society of Homeopaths member, says she has used CEASE therapy if parents have requested it. Smits' book, she says, is written for lay people, who then look for a therapist.

'I would never promise to cure anything. I do think autism can be treated. It can be improved,' she said. Children often had gut disorders, she said, adding: 'I'm not a gut specialist. That's what Andrew Wakefield was working on.'

She claimed: 'There are a lot of scientists finding similar results to his.'

While the causes of autistic spectrum disorder are unclear, she says on her website that 'ASD is often linked to vaccine damage' and asks parents to fill in a questionnaire 'if you feel you or your children have been damaged by vaccines'.

Asked about the CEASE theory that fever and diarrhoea help expel toxins, she said: 'Generally speaking in homeopathy, discharge can be a good

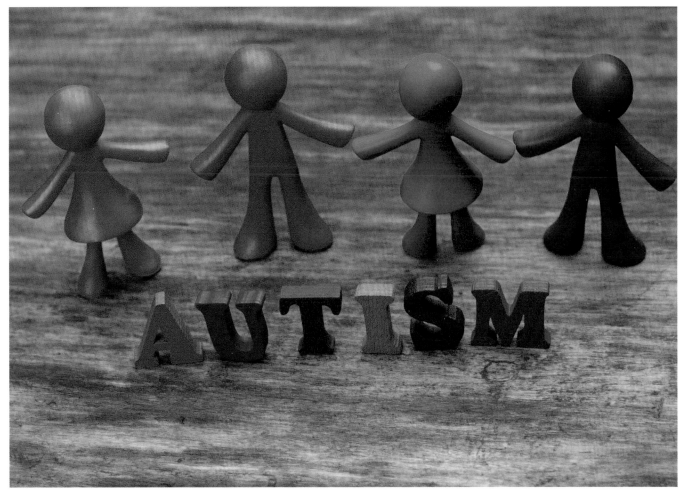

thing. If you have infected wounds, you want the pus to come out. If you have diarrhoea you want it to come out rather than be constipated.' A child must not be allowed to become dehydrated, however.

Smits, the creator of CEASE therapy, wrote in his book that 'all kinds of detoxification reactions may occur' as a result of the treatment. Most common is fever, he said, which 'should not be treated with medication, as it is a healthy reaction of the organism and not a disease! . . . Eliminations like diarrhoea, flu, expectoration, and bad-smelling and cloudy urine should also be left alone, because they are a part of the healing process.'

One child he treated had diarrhoea that 'relieved his system so much that his autism almost disappeared instantly'. After 10 days, however, his mother was so concerned that she took him to the doctor, who gave him immodium to stop the diarrhoea.

'Almost immediately the child had a setback and became autistic as before. The diarrhea was a perfect detoxification for his bowels and brain. Neither the doctor not the mother understood this, and the medication interfered with the progress of the cure,' claimed Smits.

Ursula Kraus-Harper, a member of the Society of Homeopaths, told *The Guardian* she has used CEASE therapy since attending a seminar with Smits in 2010 but that she uses it in conjunction with classical homeopathy. Children started improving after a certain set of detoxes, she said. She did not believe homeopathy was a cure, however.

She said she was not against vaccination, but said 'vaccines can be a problem and so can medical drugs. That is more and more accepted by everybody who is not blinded by drug-driven medicine.' She denied CEASE put children at risk. 'Tell me of one child, one person that has died

from high doses of vitamin C,' she said. 'When the body has had too much of it, it will produce diarrhoea; then you lower the dose and the diarrhoea will stop.'

The Labour MP Barry Sheerman, who chaired the cross-party Westminster Commission on Autism, condemned the claims of CEASE therapists to cure the disorder. 'There is support and much we can do but there are no cures and if someone says so, show me the evidence,' he said.

27 April 2018

⇨ The above information is reprinted with kind permission from *The Guardian*. Please visit www.theguardian.com for further information.

© *2018 Guardian News and Media Limited*

Kefir – the 'feel good' drink

By Dr Laura Wyness (PhD, MSc, BSc, RNutr), Listed Nutritionist

What is it?

Kefir is a fermented milk drink that seems to be gaining popularity in the UK due to its high probiotic content and beneficial effect on gut health and digestion. The drink originated from parts of Eastern Europe and Southwest Asia with the name coming from the Turkish word Keyif, which means 'feeling good' after eating.

How's it made?

Kefir is most commonly made with pasteurised whole, semi-skimmed or skimmed cow's milk, although goats, sheep, buffalo or camel milk may also be used. It's made by adding kefir grains to the milk and leaving it to ferment, usually for about 24 hours. The grains are then removed from the liquid and can be used again.

Now it's probably worth pointing out that the kefir 'grains' are not cereal grains but they are in fact cultures of bacteria and yeast and are white-ish, gel-like irregular shapes of variable size from about 0.3cm to 3.5cm in diameter. The grains actually look more like a cauliflower head.

Is it tasty?

The kefir drink tastes a bit sour, similar to a runny yoghurt and a bit fizzy. This is due to the main products of kefir fermentation – lactic acid, ethanol and carbon dioxide (CO_2). Taste is personal, so you'll need to try it for yourself! If you've not had kefir before, try a small amount at first as kefir can cause some intestinal cramping and constipation if your gut is not used to so much probiotic activity and diversity.

Is it nutritious?

In terms of the nutritional content, it can vary widely and depends on

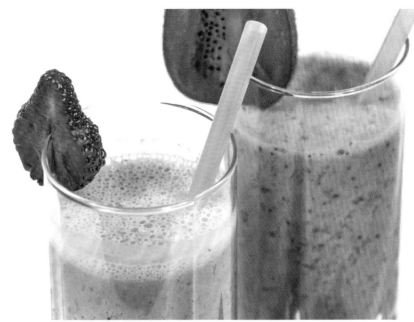

the type of milk used, the origin and composition of the kefir grains, the time and temperature of fermentation and the storage conditions. A glass of kefir (175ml) provides around:

Energy	104 kcal (433kJ)*
Fat	3-6g*
Carbohydrate	7-8g*
Protein	about 6g
Calcium	187mg
Riboflavin (Vitamin B2)	0.3mg
Vitamin B12	0.33mg
Phosphorus	148mg
Magnesium	19mg

* (depending on the type of milk used)

Dairy free versions of kefir can also be made with coconut water or other plant liquids, although these will not have the same nutrient profile as dairy-based kefir.

Kefir has a high probiotic activity and contains a wide variety of bioactive compounds, including organic acids, peptides and kefiran (the main polysaccharide in kefir) that all add to its health benefits.

What are the benefits of drinking kefir?

Kefir is packed with probiotics – more, in terms of both the number and variety than yoghurt and many other fermented foods. We now know that lots of probiotics of a wide diversity is key to a healthy and happy gut. With the increasing awareness and research on gut health, kefir could provide an attractive and beneficial probiotic drink for many consumers.

Scientific studies support the health benefits of kefir such as improved digestion and tolerance to lactose, anti-bacterial effect, reducing cholesterol levels, improving blood sugar levels, helping to control blood pressure, an anti-inflammatory effect, antioxidant activity, anti-cancer activity, anti-allergenic activity and healing effects. However, there is still a need for better understanding of the composition of kefir, more research to understand the physiological benefits and how kefir works in our body, and better quality human trials with adequate sample size and study duration.

How can I make it?

You can make kefir yourself at home using the traditional method which involves milk inoculation with a variable amount of kefir grains and leaving it to ferment for 18–24 hours at around 20–25°C. The grains are then sieved and can be used again, and the kefir drink is stored at 4°C.

On a larger scale, the 'Russian method' or the commercial process using pure cultures can be used. The use of commercial cultures can standardise the commercial production of kefir and the end drink could have a shelf-life of 28 days. Kefir produced with grains should be consumed within three to 12 days. It's also worth noting that the commercially produced kefir-type drink may not have the same beneficial and probiotic properties present in traditional kefir.

What kefir-based products are available?

There is increasing interest in the development of functional foods that will benefit health and help prevent diseases, and new kefir products seem to be appearing on the market. One of the largest kefir companies is Lifeway, which has products available in the USA, Canada and the UK. Other companies include Evolve Kefir and Wallaby Yoghurt Company with a range of kefir drinks, yoghurts, cheese and ice-cream.

27 June 2017

⇨ The above information is reprinted with kind permission from Nutritionist Resource. Please visit www.nutritionist-resource. org.uk for further information.

© 2018 Nutritionist Resource

Why traditional healers could have a role to play in fighting HIV   THE CONVERSATION

An article from **The Conversation.**

By Ryan G. Wagner, Research Fellow, MRC/Wits Rural Public Health & Health Transitions Research Unit (Agincourt), University of Witwatersrand and Carolyn Audet, Assistant Professor in the Department of Health Policy at the Vanderbilt Institute of Global Health, Vanderbilt University

Many cultures and societies throughout the world turn to traditional healers to find out why they are ill and to seek treatment. In many settings, including sub-Saharan Africa, traditional healers are often called on to provide cures for various ailments.

Seeking help from traditional healers can have a detrimental effect on a patient because it can delay them getting the care or treatment they need from health facilities. This is a particularly pertinent challenge when it comes to treating HIV because getting access to treatment as early as possible after being diagnosed has been shown to be very important. In addition, studies have shown that traditional medicine can affect the efficacy of antiretroviral treatment.

We were keen to understand how people living with HIV in rural communities in South Africa consulted traditional healers, and how this affected whether or not they sought treatment from local clinics. Our study, done in rural northeastern South Africa, has an HIV prevalence of 19.4% among adults. This is one of the highest figures in the world.

We found that some traditional healers continued to treat HIV-positive people for HIV and their associated opportunistic infections. But it also showed that they referred their patients for HIV testing at public health facilities. This suggests that they saw the value of HIV testing.

The study, undertaken in an area where the South African Government's health facilities offer free antiretroviral treatment, raises important questions about the role that traditional healers play in providing health care. It shows that working with traditional healers could lead to health care that integrates both approaches. Studies from other developing countries has shown that this can have benefits.

One, or both

People seek care from traditional healers for different reasons. Often they are able to access the traditional healer more easily than health professionals. Medication shortages at clinics and hospitals also play a role. For others there are greater cultural similarities between the traditional healers' explanation of their condition and their own understanding.

Research shows that people felt they were treated better by traditional healers than carers in the public health system.

Traditional healers and health professionals often treat patients

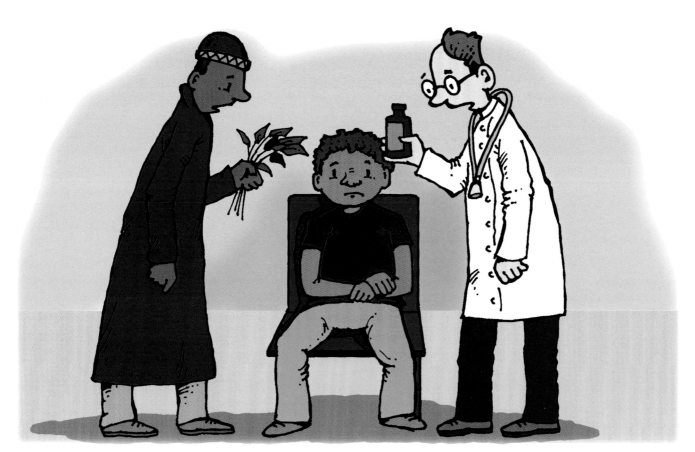

concurrently. Patients choose to use one or the other – or both. This results in a 'ping-pong' effect of patients moving between traditional healers and healthcare facilities.

There are dangers in this – using traditional medicine and ART concurrently have been shown to have negative effects in some instances.

Examples of integration

There have been attempts to incorporate traditional healers into healthcare systems. A number of projects and studies have been done in several African countries including Cameroon and Mozambique to integrate traditional healers with health professionals.

These projects have had mixed results. Traditional healers are a heterogeneous population: not all healers will make effective partners with clinicians and nurses in the healthcare system. Some healers fear losing income, others do not believe nurses and clinicians can cure all ailments and a history of distrust has damaged relationships between healers and clinicians.

But engaging healers has resulted in several successful partnerships. These have included:

⇨ Increasing traditional healers' knowledge of diseases and conditions

⇨ Reducing the delay of patients getting care from health facilities for time-sensitive conditions

⇨ Improving the relationship between healers and health professionals

In Mozambique, ongoing research with traditional healers has resulted in the development of a referral-back-referral system. Traditional healers refer patients to a clinic to be tested for HIV and other common ailments. The patients then return to the traditional healer with a clear referral of the clinic's findings.

Our research shows similar results. About 85% of traditional healers referred their patients for HIV testing at public health facilities before initiating traditional care. And traditional healers used a patient's CD4 count as a threshold to determine whether further traditional treatment should be offered.

Keep the ball rolling

Great progress has been made in managing the HIV/AIDS pandemic. Key to this success has been ensuring people are tested and then introduced to drug regimens as soon as possible.

While the push for a functional cure and more effective treatment and treatment delivery systems are important, so too is understanding and mitigating barriers to existing care. Keeping a cautious, yet open mind to the complementary role that traditional healers can play could help further reduce – and support the ultimate end of – the HIV/AIDS pandemic.

30 November 2017

⇨ The above information is reprinted with kind permission from *The Conversation*. Please visit www. theconversation.com for further information.

Key facts

- There is an important difference between a complementary therapy and an alternative therapy. (page 1)
  - A complementary therapy means you can use it alongside your conventional medical treatment. It may help you to feel better and cope better with your cancer and treatment. (page 1)
  - An alternative therapy is generally used instead of conventional medical treatment. (page 1)
- Chinese herbal medicine is one of the great herbal systems of the world, with an unbroken tradition going back to the 3rd century BC. (page 4)
- Homeopathy is a complementary or alternative medicine (CAM). This means that homeopathy is different from treatments that are part of conventional Western medicine in important ways. (page 9)
- Teachers of the Alexander Technique believe it helps get rid of tension in your body and relieves problems such as back pain, neck ache, sore shoulders and other musculoskeletal problems. (page 11)
- Reiki, pronounced 'ray-key', is a system of energy healing originating from Japan. The word reiki itself translates to 'universal life energy' and is based on the belief that life energy flows through all living things. When this energy becomes disrupted or blocked, it is believed that stress and disease follow. (page 12)
- Herbal medicines are plant-based medicines made from differing combinations of plant parts, e.g. leaves, flowers or roots. Each part can have different medicinal uses and the many types of chemical constituents require different extraction methods. Both fresh and dried plant matter are used, depending on the herb. (page 14)
- Doctors in China have been pushing needles into patients' skin, supposedly to restore the flow of healing 'qi energy', for more than 4,000 years. (page 16)
- An overview of studies (a meta analysis) published in 2012 suggested that around half of people with cancer use some sort of complementary therapy at some time during their illness. (page 18)
- Period pain, or dysmenorrhea, is a condition affecting up to 95 per cent of menstruating women. (page 21)
- According to analysis of spoken conversations, approximately 80–90 spoken words each day – 0.5% to 0.7% of all words – are swear words, with usage varying from between 0% to 3.4%. In comparison, first-person plural pronouns (we, us, our) make up 1% of spoken words. (page 23)
  - The first person to swear on British national television – Kenneth Tynan (1965). (page 23)

- Every year there are around one million hospital admissions of children under 15, many of them serious and extended. With their tiny team of just 25 giggle doctors, Theodora Children's Charity is able to visit 33,000 of these children each year. (page 24)
  - In a typical visit a giggle doctor may see 25 children, spending about ten minutes with each one. In a year one giggle doctor will visit over 1,000 children. (page 24)
- The word trepanation comes from the Greek trypanon, meaning a borer. The earliest known trepanned skulls date from around 10,000 BCE, and come from North Africa. (page 25)
- The NHS currently spends £92,412 a year on the natural 'treatment', which uses highly diluted doses of natural substances that some claim help the body heal itself. (page 29)
- When tested under rigorous conditions – when neither the patient nor the doctor knows whether they're using homeopathy or not until all of the tests are done – homeopathy has shown to work no better than a sugar pill. (page 30)
  - The homeopathy industry is worth around £40 million in the UK, and around €400 million in both France and Germany. (page 30)
  - Homeopathic pills are being sold at a cost of around £5.95 for less than 20g of sugar pills. Without any active ingredient, that ultimately amounts to a lot of money for not a lot of sugar. (page 30)
  - In the UK, the NHS spends an estimated £4 million every year on homeopathy. (page 30)
- Prescription antibiotics, such as penicillin, have helped people to recover from otherwise fatal diseases and conditions since the 1940s. (page 31)
  - According to the NHS, one in ten people experiences side effects that harm the digestive system after taking antibiotics. Around one in 15 people are allergic to this type of medication. (page 31)
- More than 120 homeopaths in the UK are offering a 'cure' for autism that involves supposedly detoxing children of the vaccines and antibiotics held responsible for the condition. (page 35)
- Northeastern South Africa, has an HIV prevalence of 19.4% among adults. This is one of the highest figures in the world. (page 38)
  - Some traditional healers continued to treat HIV-positive people for HIV and their associated opportunistic infections. But it also showed that they referred their patients for HIV testing at public health facilities. This suggests that they saw the value of HIV testing. (page 38)

Acupuncture

An ancient practice which involves inserting sterile needles into strategic points on the human body with the aim of relieving pain and other negative symptoms.

Aromatherapy

Aromatherapy utilises scented 'essential oils', which practitioners claim will induce certain moods or promote good health (e.g. calming/relaxation). They can be inhaled, used as a massage oil or occasionally ingested. There are over 400 different essential oils and they are extracted from plants all over the world. Popular oils used include camomile, lavender, rosemary and tea tree.

Chiropractic

A system of complementary medicine based on the diagnosis and manipulative treatment of misalignments of the joints, especially those of the spinal column, which are believed to cause other disorders by affecting the nerves, muscles, and organs.

Complementary and alternative medicine (CAM)

CAM includes a wide range of therapies and practices that are outside the mainstream of medicine: for example, homeopathy, herbal remedies, acupuncture, reflexology, reiki and traditional Chinese medicine. Complementary medicine uses therapies that work alongside conventional medicine. Alternative medicine includes treatments that are not currently considered part of evidence-based Western medicine. However, as the distinction between the two is not clear-cut, the term complementary and alternative medicine (CAM) is now widely used to include both approaches. The effectiveness of some forms of CAM is often hotly debated.

Homeopathy

A form of alternative medicine in which practitioners use highly diluted substances to treat their patients. The thinking behind this practice is that when substances known to cause certain symptoms are delivered to patients exhibiting those same symptoms in a highly diluted form, the substances will be effective as a treatment. According to the Society of Homeopaths' website, a homeopathic remedy of 30C contains less than one part per million of the original substance. While practitioners and patients are vocal supporters of the benefits of homeopathy, its critics claim that there is a lack of scientific and clinical evidence to support it and that it offers little more than a placebo effect.

Massage therapy

A 'therapeutic touch' which can be used for health benefits, such as helping people relax, making people feel energised, relieving tension or helping ease muscle pain/stiffness. There are many different massage styles and techniques which involve the use of a varying number of movements and pressures on different parts of the body. Some of the most common types of massage are Swedish massage, deep tissue massage and Indian head massage – each have their own specialist techniques that tackle different ailments.

Osteopathy

A system of complementary medicine involving the treatment of medical disorders through the manipulation and massage of the skeleton and musculature.

Placebo

A placebo is a substance administered to patients containing no active ingredients: for example, a sugar pill or saline solution. However, the patient taking the placebo is led to believe that it is a medicine which will have a positive effect on certain symptoms they are displaying. The 'placebo effect' refers to an improvement in symptoms brought about by a patient's belief that the inactive substance they are taking will cure or improve their illness. Critics of certain types of alternative medicine, for example homeopathy, believe that the treatments given to patients by practitioners are little more than placebos.

Yoga

With historical origins in ancient Indian philosophy, yoga aims to transform the mind and body through physical, mental and spiritual disciplines. With regular practise, the exercise of yoga is meant to bring health benefits such as increased energy levels, relief from muscle pain and stiffness, and improved circulation.

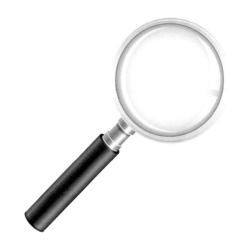

Assignments

Brainstorming

⇨ Brainstorm what you know about complementary and alternative medicine.

- What is complementary medicine?

- What is alternative medicine?

- What is herbal medicine?

- What is homeopathy?

- What does the term 'placebo' mean?

Research

⇨ Do some research into the types of complementary and alternative medicines available. Make a list of at least five of the ones you come across, giving a short description of each. Share with the rest of your class.

⇨ Conduct a survey amongst your family and friends to find out if any of them have used alternative medicines and if so, which ones. You should ask at least six questions and write a short report on your findings.

⇨ In pairs, do some research into the differences between complementary and alternative medicines. You should consider why someone might decide to use these instead of conventional medicine. Write some notes on your findings and feedback to your class.

⇨ Do some research into herbal medicine. What is a herbalist? You should look into what conditions can be treated with herbal medicine and how effective it might be. Write a short report on your findings and share with your class.

⇨ Do some research into the health benefits of honey. Find out the origins of the use of honey for treatment of ailments and what it is used for today.

Design

⇨ Imagine you work for a company that manufactures herbal medicines. Design a poster to advertise your products.

⇨ Design a fitness tracker. What will it be called?

⇨ Design a leaflet informing people of the different types of alternative therapies that are available. You should make a list and write a one-paragraph description of each therapy. You should also give some information as to where people could access the different therapies.

⇨ Choose one of the articles in this book and create an illustration to highlight the key themes/messages of your chosen article.

⇨ Read the article on page 24 about 'giggle doctors' and design a poster advertising their services which is to be displayed in hospitals.

Oral

⇨ As a class read the article on page 16 'Pains and needles: brain scans point to hidden effects of acupuncture'. Discuss the use of acupuncture and if you think it is genuinely effective or just 'placebo'.

⇨ In pairs, discuss the use of alternative medicine versus conventional medicine. One of you should argue in favour of alternative medicine and the other against. Then swap roles.

⇨ On page 24 it says 'trained and paid to go round hospitals to cheer up children with music and laughter'. Divide the class into two halves. Each half should write their own one-minute repertoire aimed at cheering up a sick child. Then each half should perform for the other half of the class.

⇨ In small groups, choose one of the illustrations from the book and consider what message your chosen picture is trying to get across. How does it support, or add to, the points made in the accompanying article? Do you think it is successful?

⇨ In groups, prepare a PowerPoint presentation showing the different types of alternative therapies which are available. You should give some information about each therapy and the benefits of using such treatments.

Reading/writing

⇨ Write a one-paragraph definition of aromotherapy and compare it to a classmate's.

⇨ Write a one-paragraph definition of hypnotherapy and compare it to a classmate's.

⇨ Write a short article about complementary therapies. You can use the article on page 6 to help you.

⇨ Write an essay about homeopathy. It should cover at least two sides of A4. You should consider what it is used to treat and how safe it is. You should end your essay by giving your views on this treatment.

⇨ Write an article exploring the use of acupuncture for relieving period pain. Read the article on page 21 for help.

⇨ Write an article for your student newspaper arguing that homeopathy has no place within the National Health Service. You will need to support your argument with evidence, informing readers of the costs involved and the effectiveness of the treatments.

⇨ Write an open letter to GPs advocating the use of homeopathy. Use your letter to highlight its benefits and try to persuade them to use this form of natural treatment.

Acknowledgements

The publisher is grateful for permission to reproduce the material in this book. While every care has been taken to trace and acknowledge copyright, the publisher tenders its apology for any accidental infringement or where copyright has proved untraceable. The publisher would be pleased to come to a suitable arrangement in any such case with the rightful owner.

Images

All images courtesy of iStock except pages 5, 7, 13, 15, 20, 22, 28, 29 and 37: Pixabay

Illustrations

Don Hatcher: pages 23 & 39. Simon Kneebone: pages 16 & 32. Angelo Madrid: pages 8 & 27.

Additional acknowledgements

With thanks to the Independence team: Shelley Baldry, Danielle Lobban, Jackie Staines and Jan Sunderland.

Tina Brand

Cambridge, October 2018